No Duty to Retreat

The Stories of Tourette's Disease and Asperger's Autism

Most Reverend E. Antonio Hernández, O.M.D.

PublishAmerica
Baltimore

First printing

ISBN: 1-59286-926-2
PUBLISHED BY PUBLISHAMERICA, LLLP
www.publishamerica.com
Baltimore

Printed in the United States of America

For Chris, my eternal Boo
and
for my beloved mother
and
for my beloved grandmother

SECTION I:

TOURETTE'S DISEASE, HISTORY AND TICS

Foreword

Our world is full of so many types of people that we tend to over-type too often. Some people are ill, and then of course they must be typed. Some people twitch, make noises and mimic sounds or voices. They are typed as having Tourette Syndrome. Some rock back and forth, never uttering a word, seemingly unreachable. They are typed as autistic. Some are consumed by horrible or persistent thoughts and ideas, imprisoned by routines and rituals. They are typed as obsessive compulsive. Some are eccentric and appear to us as behaving totally inappropriately. It's anybody's guess how they are typed. Some, most in fact, exhibit all these characteristics, and no one is yet certain how to type them. All are valuable, all have something to teach, something to give. This book is about such people.

Tourette's Disease, popularly known as Tourette's Syndrome (TS), is a neurological muscular movement disorder, classed in medical books alongside its cousin Parkinson's Disease. It is a disease comprised of tics: any behavior, activity or emotion that is sudden and involuntary. It sometimes features a whole spectrum of mimicry. Asperger's autism, popularly known as Asperger's Syndrome, was studied and delineated in 1944 by Dr. Hans Asperger of Vienna. At the same time, Dr. Leo Kanner of Johns Hopkins was studying deeply disabled, retarded individuals; Dr. Kanner also chose the label autism, today known as Early Infantile Autism.

Asperger's autism is classified as a mild, high function (HF) form of autism (also abbreviated as HFA) that includes a triad of disabilities: social, communicative, and imaginative. It frequently includes very high intelligence and multiple talents. Like Tourette's Disease, it includes tics and mimicry. Obsessive Compulsive Disorder (OCD) is considered an anxiety disorder. It is characterized by two symptomologies: obsessions, which are mental perseverations, and compulsions, which are virtually like tics. Compulsions are involuntary and complicated behaviors—behaviors which were once believed to afford relief to the OCD sufferer. In addition, OCD may feature a sub-category of symptoms known as impulsive. Tourettic and autistic behaviors are very common in OCD; OCD is commonly seen in both TS and AS.

Please note that the book is in two major sections. Section I will introduce Tourette's Disease and its history, going on to examine Tourette's major feature, tics. Section II will be devoted to Asperger's Autism, autism in general, their histories and related topics not otherwise covered. I have deliberately left Section I leaning more or less exclusively toward Tourette's Disease, so as to be able to expand and "breathe" a bit more in Section II.

Autism, Tourette's Disease and OCD all share a part of my life: I have been diagnosed with all three. Despite this and a few other conditions, which shall presently be addressed, my life has been mostly full and relatively happy. After decades of research and dead ends, I finally fathomed the deep mysteries of my life—the dark, tormented, miserable side of my life. When I did uncover all the secrets, my life was dark, tormented, miserable no more.

This book tells a story more than anything else: the story of how these illnesses were discovered and how I discovered them in myself, the story of how the illnesses have touched my life, how I studied and learned about every detail of these illnesses, and the story of how we can move on, understanding and coping. It is a story of hope, of answers, of resources and of theories. I offer it to one and all, in the hope that it will assist, guide, and teach—just as I was assisted, guided and taught so many years ago. I hope that this book is accepted as a cherished gift, a memento of that journey I undertook years ago. Think of this book, even through the difficult parts, as a long letter to a dear friend. As you read it, consider yourself the friend to whom it was addressed.

Prologue-In-Parts

Reality is devoid of any intrinsic identity that can ever be captured by any single proposition...

-His Holiness XIVth Dalai Lama

When I was around five, my parents and I were waiting in the customs office at Laredo, Texas. We were on our way into Mexico, where I spent all my childhood summers. My attention was fixed on a young girl, a beatnik type. As I recall she looked rather radiant, with long reddish-brown hair in braids, a billowy paisley blouse and slacks. She was gyrating in her seat, rocking, flapping her hands as if they were burnt, and repeating an odd phrase over and over. My parents noticed her and said something about "that crazy girl."

But being a child I knew better: somehow I sensed that she was really just existing on her own plane. I named her the Shaky Lady, and she has a permanent place in my memory. After seeing the Shaky Lady, many more such people seemed to pop up, every place I went. They all received affectionate, childish nicknames. It is wonderful to have the mind of a child. What I did not come to realize until recently is that they all probably suffered from the same disease: TOURETTE'S SYNDROME. I find it preferable to call this condition rightly: Tourette's Disease. This book will use various names for it, but do not be mistaken. Tourette's is a disease.

Some years ago I was suddenly reminded of several kids I knew in grade school who also showed evidence of Tourette's Syndrome, and I even recalled a few teachers whom I suspected. Suddenly, within these last few years, I began seeing it all over the place. At one point in my life I was stunned to count more than a dozen people I know personally who showed TS symptoms; scattered among them are more members of my immediate family than I can count. In considering this, I knew that the Tourette prevalence statistics were very wrong. At the time, doctors counted an average of one in ten thousand afflicted with TS. Later, I began seeing eerie similarities with TS in people with autism.

My first job was in a state home devoted to the care of profoundly retarded and autistic adults. It gave me the opportunity to work with and care for autistics of all types. Imagine my shock when I was diagnosed with a form of autism, called Asperger's Syndrome, some years ago. I then discovered that autism features very strongly in many Tourette cases—and that autistics manifest many tourettic symptoms. I took another good look at my family and discovered seven members who show signs of mild autism.

Since this book hopes to introduce you fully to Tourette's Disease and mild autism from a sufferer's viewpoint, I will again state officially: I suffer from Tourette's Disease, Obsessive Compulsive Disorder, Attention Deficit Hyperactive Disorder (ADHD, falling into the general category of Attention Deficit Syndromes, or ADS), along with several other learning disabilities, and Asperger's Syndrome, which I call Asperger's autism, a very high function form of autism.

My diagnoses were made at different times some years ago; the first diagnosis, OCD, was made in the early 1980's. My life had been one long, seemingly endless search for the truth about myself. Years of pain, fear, anger and the feeling of insanity took their toll, but I persevered. Tourette's Disease was diagnosed in March of 1994. The last diagnosis, which had been noticed very early but had never been determined, is Asperger's autism. This diagnosis was made at the end of January, 2000.

You will note that references to autism in general are laced throughout this book, right next to the facts about Tourette's Disease. I did this for a purpose: to argue what is admittedly an educated guess, but I think a very good guess. My guess is that Asperger's autism is probably much more common than anyone thinks, and I believe it to be one and the same as TS and OCD. AS patients are usually very gifted and intelligent, seem basically normal, and show few autistic features. AS has been seen frequently in combination with TS; some experts are suggesting a common gene for AS, TS, OCD, ADS and even addictive behaviors.

We shall explore this genetic link later, along with my theory that all these conditions may represent a single, as yet unidentified neurological disease that can manifest, as Dr. Oliver Sacks discovered, in infinite ways. It's very beautiful the way nature attempts to balance a person; my troubles with autism are counteracted by tourettic symptoms. My ADHD (if that's what it is) is sometimes helped by my obsessive compulsive traits. TS, AS, OCD, ADHD! What an alphabet soup I've got going!

One final thing: my doctors have urged me to keep quiet about the autism (so much for my taking advice!). For one thing, they tell me, no one really knows much about it, and I agree. Though many experts have a clear grip on the general symptomology, many doctors are at a standstill whether or not Asperger's is even autism at all. This puzzles me; I see no barrier preventing AS from being rightly called autism. Also, my doctors have pointed out that sharing this facet of my troubles could label me in a negative way. I don't know why; it's an individual's own problem if he chooses to be negative about illness.

Dr. Tony Attwood, one of the experts on Asperger's autism, says it's easier to just choose the label "Asperger's Syndrome," thus avoiding the autism stigma. I can't say I altogether agree with his reasoning, though I agree that a label should be chosen appropriately. One of my former doctors told me I don't show any sign of it at all. These asides are nothing but balderdash and horsefeathers. There will be more about this later. Please remember that generally, when you see the word "autism" in the text, I am referring to Asperger's high functioning autism (AS or HF autism) unless otherwise stated.

Please, sit back and relax. Enjoy this book, even if some parts appear a little frightening. My earlier manuscript was rejected by a prominent publishing house on the shaky grounds that it was just too scary. I have a pet phrase I use in my practice as a doctor of Oriental medicine: We'll get through this!

Prologue II:
The Wrong Stuff

Men in long battle are not normal men.
-John Steinbeck

"I have Tourette's Disease." There seems to be something quasi-mystical, something terrible, in saying that—sort of like the feeling many experience when hearing, "I was in Viet Nam." My diagnosis wasn't made until 1994, so I hadn't begun researching Tourette Syndrome until prior to the end of 1993, when I did intense research and a complete medical history of myself using lists of Tourette guidelines as a sort of map. After learning as much as possible, I quite by chance encountered a book still in use today that really surprised me. It had alot of information about the 19th century history of the illness, but it also contained rather blaring mistakes written by the editing physicians who compiled it.

In reading this book, Advances in Neurology Vol. 35 (1982), the first chapter of which deals with Tourette Syndrome, it became clear to me that advances in its study have been incredibly slow. It surprises me to see that the original and very accurate ideas about it are totally neglected in most of the modern literature; the Advances editors' mistakes, repeated again and again, are eloquent testimony of this. As a TS patient suffering from myriad disabilities, I noted many interesting 19th century clinical observations in the text that could help modern researchers if they would only pay attention. The observations are things that I know from my own experience.

The first chapter of the textbook is entitled "Gilles de la Tourette on Tourette Syndrome," by Drs. Goetz and Klawans. It contains the significant information discovered by de la Tourette himself, which I would like to summarize here. It is probable that few people are familiar with Dr. de la Tourette's original discoveries, delineation, and the work that led to his research. It is the most highly valuable of all the Tourette literature, containing the efforts of the first people of the modern era to seriously research Tourette's Syndrome medically.

Before summarizing the events directly related to Tourette's original research, I would like to mention the research that was done regarding the involuntary movement found in all normal, healthy human beings. It is seminal research that was done, curiously, at the same time as the Tourette research first began: 1812.

In 1812 a famous French chemist, Chevreul, experimented with the "magic pendulum" to see why it moved. He discovered that the movement is caused by the pendulum-holder's own involuntary muscular movement, brought on by autosuggestion or outside suggestion. Not until 1833, at the urging of Ampère, did Chevreul publish his findings, in the form of an open letter addressed to Ampère. In 1852, English physiologist William Carpenter coined the term "ideomotor" to define the subtle tic activity already described by Chevreul—which may fairly be labeled the "Chevreul Effect." Then in 1853 the French Academy of Science appointed Chevreul head of a three-man committee to formally study and define this neuro-muscular movement phenomenon.

Chevreul published the formal paper on involuntary movements in 1854. We shall have the chance to learn all about Chevreul and his work in the upcoming Chevreul chapter. What is odd is that in spite of the importance of Chevreul's work, his being a contemporary colleague of the great French scientists of the 19th century, and his great fame, there is no mention of him or his works in any of the original Tourette literature. I could not even find proof that any of the scientists knew or heard of Chevreul—other than to note that Chevreul was widely known throughout Europe. What is even stranger about this evident ignorance of Chevreul is that he continued as a prominent scientist until his death—at the age of 103.

Now to proceed with the summary of Tourette research history: in 1825 the famous French neurologist Dr. Jean-Marc Itard published a paper on one Madame la Marquise de Dampierre, a French aristocrat. Dr. Itard is famous for bringing into society a supposed "wild boy"; he taught the boy and helped him become more human. Ironically, the boy likely suffered from autism. Anyhow, the noblewoman displayed an alarming array of Tourette symptoms;

she has achieved a fame of sorts as the first contemporarily studied TS patient. Dr. Itard, not Dr. de la Tourette, was thus the first to write clinically about the illness.

This same year Dr. Jean-Martin Charcot, a teacher of Tourette and Freud, took over the treatment of this poor lady and also published work about her condition. Sometime in 1861 a Dr. Armand Trousseau wrote a thorough paper on vocal Tourette Syndrome symptoms, which he differentiated from better-known choreaic symptoms. This detail fascinates us because it came after the publication of Chevreul's formal paper on "normal" involuntary movements, but again, there is no reference to what Chevreul wrote. I suspect this is because the earliest work on Tourette symptoms was for the most part in the realm of medical research on chorea. Chevreul was not a doctor but a chemist, and he was writing not about diseases but about normal behavioral phenomena.

In 1884 Dr. Georges Gilles de la Tourette published a preliminary paper on his eight TS patients who had previously been in the care of Dr. Charcot. Essentially, Itard and Charcot handed the cases to Tourette. Tourette was considered a brilliant clinician at the Salpétrière Hospital in France, and was thought by all to be the best scientist for these cases. Tourette was young—a great plus. It was Charcot who generously christened the disease "Tourette's Syndrome," though Tourette himself called it a disease of "false chorea."

Another oddity I want point out is the time discrepancy between the works: it is in 1812 that Chevreul more or less secretly researches involuntary movement in normal people; it is in the 1820's that the first Tourette symptoms are addressed; it is in 1833 that Chevreul publishes his first work on involuntary movement, but it is not until 1884 that de la Tourette publishes his first work on Tourette Disease. The only other work extant between these two periods of time consists of mere references to choreaic movements, and even these occur only after the middle of the century.

In 1885 de la Tourette published his major paper on TS, entitled "Study of a Neurologic Condition Characterized by Motor Incoördination [this was Tourette's term for tics] Accompanied by Echolalia and Coprolalia (Jumping, Latah, Myriachit)." Dr. Tourette begins by citing one Dr. Bouteille, who was the first to do a serious paper on chorea, entitled "Traité de la Chorée" ["Tract on Chorea"]. Chorea is defined as any disease of the nervous system that involves short, jerky, involuntary movements, and this illness was being thoroughly researched at this time.

Dr. Tourette is careful to mention that Bouteille was the first to properly differentiate choreaic neurological diseases and among the first to mention, in passing, some symptoms of what came to be known as Tourette Syndrome: "I use [Bouteille wrote] the name pseudo-chorea or false chorea (choreés fausses) to distinguish those different nervous, spasmodic, convulsive, or hysteric afflictions which *do not show the characteristic symptoms of true chorea, the only resemblance between them and chorea being facial grimacing and involuntary movements.*" [Italics mine.]

Tourette points out that if this important sentence had been scrutinized more carefully and then followed up, there would have been less subsequent confusion about Tourette's Syndrome. In Tourette's day there was not yet even a partial description of TS anywhere in the literature, other than the rather thin but seminal work of Chevreul, Itard and Charcot.

The worst impasse, prior to Tourette's studies, was that doctors were able to do nothing more than compare TS patients to chorea patients and note the pronounced differences—and this thanks only to Bouteille and Trousseau. Doctors had been making serious comparisons only since Itard's work was published, but at least at this particular time there were no drastic or damaging attempts at treating Tourette Syndrome. Nor was there any mislabeling, all of which is more than we can claim in our own time.

In his paper, Tourette outlines the next important step in the delineation of TS. Going back to 1880, an American doctor, George Beard, presented a paper entitled "The Jumping Frenchmen." These Frenchmen, called "Jumpers," were apparently TS sufferers, who were living in Maine and Canada. There were fifty sufferers in all, and an outstanding symptom they manifested was to involuntarily obey any random command. Dr. Beard had also said it would be extremely dangerous to startle these people if they had an axe or hammer in hand, demonstrating as they did a violent startle-response. Next, in 1884, a Dr. J. A. O'Brien also reported TS among Malaysians, which they called "Latah."

It was again during that miracle year, 1884, that another vital paper was published. In *La Medicina Contemporanea* (that means "Contemporary Medicine"—sorry, I do not know why the title of this report is in Spanish), another American, Dr. William Hammond, published a paper about reports received from American naval officers sailing near Siberia. The sailors had seen Siberians afflicted with TS (in Siberian it is called "Myriachit"). The captain of the ship reported that his Siberian steward also manifested this disease, to the extent that the other crew members would say and do ridiculous things in his presence just to watch him involuntarily imitate them.

The American naval officers had received reports directly from Siberians that TS was very common in areas of Siberia, especially where the winters were harshest. (So common was the affliction that it even generated a centuries-old myth, that in northeastern Siberia there was a village of werewolves.) This is eerily confirmed in a way when we consider the many TS sufferers who complain that cold weather makes tics worse. Siberia also brings to mind Peter the Great, who was very seriously afflicted with TS. Dr. Tourette makes clear that, upon careful review of all the materials, the French Jumping, Malaysian Latah and Siberian Myriachit were one and the same disease: "his" disease! Amazingly, to this very day "Jumping," "Latah" and "Myriachit" are listed as separate disorders.

The editors of the Advances textbook have missed an important analysis here, which is worth examining. Undue reaction to startles, universal among TS sufferers, and the not so common obedience of sudden commands, is the primary feature of Jumping and Myriachit. Latah demonstrates intense, almost violent tics of mimicry. If the experts are unwilling to consider a Tourette Syndrome spectrum, then of course they will describe Jumping, Myriachit and Latah as separate disorders. What surprises me is that they do precisely this. It's the same as the experts refusing to acknowledge the milder forms of autism in spite of the proof.

As I've written, all TS patients experience symptoms of these three "disorders." I have experienced them, to the letter, and it is indeed dangerous for anyone to startle me at any time. What Dr. Tourette observed that interested him was the total loss of control the patients exhibited in reaction to being startled or overstimulated. This he observed in every single one of his own patients. There is a lesson here about attributing too much to the symptoms themselves, or rather the behaviors, and not to the overall internal condition.

Though Myriachit, Latah and Jumping patients showed what appeared to be different symptomology than "standard" TS, it is clear that they suffered from TS, and Dr. Tourette knew this. He seems to have been unable, however, to pursue these conditions further to establish the link. I believe that he may have been satisfied to simply classify Jumping, Latah and Myriachit under the TS heading and leave it at that. Too, he saw many TS patients, but does not seem to have treated anyone exclusively presenting symptoms of Jumping, Latah or Myriachit, so he probably concluded that the reports about these symptoms were incomplete—and perhaps redundant.

Tourette's paper then goes on to his own case descriptions, the first being the famous French noblewoman Mme. Dampièrre. Along with inheriting this famous "first patient" from Dr. Charcot, he was already seeing several new TS patients. Tourette was very excited about echolalia, the symptom of repeating words spoken by others (in some cases taking the extreme form of mimicry), and he mentions significantly that the Malaysian Latah patients, when mimicking Europeans, took on a "...new and special demeanor." This is particularly interesting, because it reflects the echophenomenal tics—which we will examine later at length—and particularly because it is a symptom present in autism as well.

Madame la Marquise de Dampièrre had coprolalia (the "swearing" tic) to endure as her most distressing symptom. She and all those around her were horrified as she echolated the most obscene and vulgar words and phrases. She also barked like a dog, twitching and casting about like a top. Tourette's other patients exhibited varying types of symptoms: he mentions with great curiosity the poor young man who, though a handsome and desirable bachelor, struggled mightily against his tics and compulsions, to the extent that he had no social life.

Dr. Tourette carefully noted the sounds made by his patients when in the midst of motor tics, and he quoted Dr. Armand Trousseau who, as mentioned, had described symptoms of TS in his 1861 paper in the Clinı́que Medicàle de l'Hotel Dieu Paris, vol. II. Dr. Trousseau, quoted by Dr. Tourette in 1885, referred to echolalic tics as "true forms of laryngeal or diaphragmatic chorea." Between 1885 and 1900, sixteen papers dealing with Tourette's Syndrome were published, though these are obscure and impossible to find today.

Today, Tourette experts do not require manifestations of echolalia for a diagnosis, as Dr. Tourette himself did. It is likely that he made echolalia a prerequisite because he was under the impression that motor and vocal tics always occur together, perhaps thinking that one caused or required the other. This is not necessarily the case but has been known to happen commonly. Occurrences of both vocal and motor tics at some point, whether simultaneous or not, are still required for a diagnosis of Tourette's Syndrome.

What is important to interject here is that the requirement for a TS diagnosis is tics manifesting at some point in life, yet doctors will not diagnose TS unless they actually see tics occurring in the patient. This is absolutely absurd, and we will see why in a later section. Suffice it to say for the moment that many Tourette patients go undiagnosed because of this grave diagnostic error.

The remainder of Dr. Tourette's paper consists mostly of opinions on the other case histories, with an emphasis on comparing them with the findings in Malaysia and Siberia. In the case descriptions, Dr. Tourette pays special attention to the manifestation of echolalia. He especially affords attention to a man who fought desperately to resist the urge to repeat the words of others. There is something about Tourette's interest in echolalia and other phonic tics that we may be overlooking. It is possible that Tourette thought the part of the brain involving language usage might be malfunctioning or damaged in cases of Tourette Syndrome, and certainly he suspected that the language center was being mightily affected.

In *Advances in Neurology*, there follows a commentary on Tourette's findings which is surprising in its inaccuracy. The editors claim, as we have already noted, that the Jumpers, Latah and Myriachit sufferers each had disorders distinct from TS. It should be clear today, as it was to Tourette, that these are not separate diseases. But let me quote from the editors' commentary:

> *Jumpers* manifest startle (stimulus-sensitive) myoclonus [a rapid, tic-like jerk of the muscles] and compulsive movements on verbal commands.... Tourette believed that the stimulus-sensitive myoclonus of latah was a form of echopraxia [mimicry of movements]. *Latah* is a continuum from mere undue excitability to startle myoclonus with echopraxia as a major feature. *Myriachit* [consists primarily of] echopraxia and echolalia. *Spontaneous tics are not seen in any of these disorders.* [Italics mine.]

What other evidence did these doctors need to realize that they were indeed discussing one and the same illness? Their own writing reveals it. Compulsive involuntary movements and tics are prominent features, as recognized even by Klawans and Goetz. Yet they separated the three conditions from Tourette Disease. It is sad that Drs. Goetz and Klawans did not more fully research and explain the Jumping, Latah or Myriachit, other than to assume they are forms of myoclonus, which is a separate movement disease, possibly related to epilepsy. If they had researched properly they would have seen that Dr. Tourette was correct.

The whole field has become a bigger, foggier mess than it was fifty years ago. Even myoclonus and its symptoms are presently in question. We have no choice but to carefully consider the work of Dr. Tourette who, as experts have refused to realize, was right all along about the vast and chameleon-like nature of tics. Even the names Tourette's Disease has borne in the past reflect a sort of chaos: Guinon's, Brissaud's II, Myospasia Impulsiva (this name sounds to me more like a car!), and Tourette's own term Choreés Fauxes, literally, "false choreas."

With the advent of the theory that Obsessive Compulsive Disorder is a form of TS, the absence of recognizable or obvious tics is really moot. However, even though obvious tics are vital to a diagnosis of TS, doctors are usually not competent enough to recognize or accept tics. Isn't that funny: they reject internal symptoms of TS and want to see tics, or else they won't diagnose TS even with a complete history. Yet these same doctors are not usually capable of seeing the subtle tics.

I can't count how many times this has happened to me, and on one occasion, a neurologist actually accused me of faking the tics (you'll read more about him later). In any case I've seen lists of the most common tics, which I think is very good information to have. I've also seen the most asinine lists, hundreds of items long, attempting to describe every possible tic. That is like trying to officially classify every "possible" type of snowflake.

It is unfairly postulated by quite a few experts that Tourette himself made too many observational errors. It seems clear that these doctors wish Tourette had made more mistakes, because they must somehow justify their own silly mistakes and inexcusable lack of progress. As a matter of fact, professional disagreement with Dr. Tourette goes all the way back to his lifetime. Freud sniffed around for some psychological origin in the tics, and almost convinced Tourette, incorrectly, that the disease lay in the purview of psychiatry. But Drs. Tourette, Trousseau, Itard and Charcot all believed TS to be purely genetic, entirely hereditary. Even so, Freud and a few others managed to halfway convince everyone that perhaps there was some psychological aspect behind some of the tics.

This is undoubtedly true in a restricted context, and it unfortunately led to ridiculous psychoanalytic interpretations of TS which persisted well into the 1970's. Even so, there were the unheeded few who insisted all along that TS is genetic. But Dr. Tourette's major findings—that TS is genetic, goes into remission with fever and does not require the presence of tics for a diagnosis—have all been shown to be true. We can forgive this great neurologist his tiny errors. But without hesitation we can rest assured that it is barbaric for the "experts" to use him not only as a kind of scapegoat, but also as an excuse to make grotesque errors of their own. And in that sense de la Tourette becomes not only their scapegoat but their Judas goat as well.

Another special point of emphasis we must consider is Dr. Tourette's own word to describe Tourette Syndrome: disease. He was under no illusions.

Tourette's "Syndrome" is a disease, and it's about time the world acknowledges this incontrovertible fact. In the Merck Manual it says that Tourette's Syndrome's nearest relative is Parkinson's Disease, since both are "neurological muscular movement diseases."

Moreover, even the 1956 edition of *Taber's Medical Dictionary* contains the entry "Tourette's Disease," though the term "syndrome" was already in wide use for other disorders. It seems we've actually been going backward and not forward in progress. What really infuriates me is the term "Tourette Disorder," as if TS were some sort of ethereal personality disorder. In fact, I would go so far as to caution against any professional who uses this term; the professional who uses this term is totally in the dark.

A syndrome is defined generally as a mysterious collection of symptoms whose origin is uncertain. Perhaps it is the uncertainty principle involved in TS that causes doctors to see it as a syndrome. Perhaps it is simply that doctors do not agree that Tourette's Disease is a disease. Perhaps it's a cover-up, as I believe, for ignorance. We know nothing about the immediate cause or causes of cancer, but cancer is most definitely not a "syndrome." Neither is diabetes, though we honestly do not know why it afflicts people.

Imagine the stupidity of writing "Cancer Syndrome" or "Diabetic Syndrome." Imagine the insult to the sufferers of these diseases by calling them "disorders." They, like Tourette's Disease, are diseases. We can admit that diseases are disorders, certainly. We can also safely say that some diseases cause syndromes. Still, it is important and life-saving to know we are dealing with diseases and not mere syndromes or disorders.

All the fancy blathering about syndromes and disorders may thrill the pants off the under-read psychiatric community. In the real world it is the difference between achieving some semblance of health and the insane asylum [see the section "Trinkle Tinkle: A Bit About Thelonious Sphere Monk"]. When I refer to my troubles in private life, I always say "Tourette's Disease." I know that Dr. Tourette and his colleagues would applaud this. As it is, I believe he's spinning around in his grave. (With Freud butting in, he was probably spinning before he ever got there.) It seems Tourette himself never had the chance to receive his proper laurels as a great doctor. Sadly for all of us, Dr. Tourette's life was cut short when, at the age of thirty-five, he was shot and killed by a psychotic woman who had been previously in the care of his hospital.

Prologue III:
A Short "Prehistory" of Tourette Syndrome

After scrutinizing the modern era's history of Tourette's Syndrome, it is natural that we might overlook past references and materials. But we should not overlook these. Tourette's Syndrome is not new; indeed, as King Solomon wrote, there is nothing new under the sun, nor is there a thought that has not been thought before. The ancient world has occasionally mentioned and mused on Tourette's Syndrome, sometimes insightfully so, sometimes frightfully so....

Dr. Oliver Sacks tells us that the first written reference to Tourette symptoms was made in ancient Greece—although I believe I've found a few references in very ancient literature from China, dating back a bit earlier, such as the so-called "Yellow Emperor's" Medical Treatise. Certainly many Chinese and Japanese Zen Buddhist masters had Tourette's Syndrome, and became famous as teachers (I'm thinking especially of the poets Han-shan from China and Reverend Ikkyu from Japan).

There is a special class of Navajo clairvoyant, called a "hand trembler." Although not medicine men, the tremblers have intense clairvoyant powers which they use to diagnose conditions or make judicial forecasts of important events. These tremblers first enter into a frenzy of motor tics before giving a reading, and their tradition dates back to the beginning of Navajo culture. A talented hand trembler is spotted in early childhood, when tics begin.

Undoubtedly, most documented cases of demonic possession over the millennia have been cases of TS. The first specific report of a TS sufferer is contained in the book *Malleus Maleficarum* ("The Witch's Hammer" or "The Hammer of Evildoing"), a tome written in 1489 by Fathers Jakob Sprenger and Hans Kraemer. The book, which is basically a Catholic handbook for identifying witches and performing exorcisms, tells of a priest with TS. It also outlines Tourette symptoms, not medically but as demonic signs. This is of some significance: TS was recognized and described, but in fanciful, metaphysical or superstitious terms. Only the Greeks distinguished themselves by proclaiming Tourette symptoms to be a sure sign of physical disease. Everyone else thought it was due to otherworldly influence, either good or evil.

It is in other more remote parts of the world that we see Tourette Disease being related to things other than mental illness. It has been revealed that Oriental populations, for some reason, exhibit a higher proportion of Tourette Disease, or at least they show it more prominently. Perhaps it's to do with how those societies handle the tourettic person. Rules of war, going back centuries and accepted today, give great deference to disabled people during wartime. It is surprising to see how people suffering specifically with Tourette's Disease were given kind consideration. Among the Indians of the United States, regardless of tribe, there was a standing order to treat such afflicted strangers with great reverence and respect. Now, where are these attitudes when we need them?

Peter the Great, the Siberian sailor who was large and fantastically handsome in his youth, first caught everyone's eye not just with his beauty but with his violent tics. He had them all over his large, muscular body. The women undoubtedly found them to be very erotic! La Marquise de Dampièrre is not the only—or the first—European patient to have become famous for having Tourette Syndrome. A 17th century French nobleman, the Prince de Conde, stuffed objects into his mouth to suppress his barking tic. Though we know little about this gentleman, this particular detail about him really tugs at the heartstrings.

Finally, we have a small list of other historical figures who are thought to have had TS, among them Samuel Johnson, Wolfgang Mozart, Ludwig van Beethoven, Modest Tchaikovsky (Piotr Illych's brother), Nikola Tesla, André Malraux and Pablo Picasso (who was thought by Jung to have been schizophrenic).

We have covered much ground, but I think it's essential to begin at the beginning, something which I haven't seen emphasized in the TS literature. Though a bit dated, the neurology text citation we examined in the Preface stands alone and as-is because I have not seen attitudes in these areas really change, as of this writing. There are no recent important sources I can find that outwardly disagree with the editorial mistakes made in Advances in Neurology.

With only two exceptions, those of Dr. Sacks and Dr. Comings, everything I read, no matter how new, actually perpetuates the mistakes. (Don't forget the medical community's motto: Rock the boat and we all die.) Dr. Tourette offers us so much more with deeper examination, and to this end I hope someday to see the publication of his complete papers on the matter.

Introduction

Form is emptiness,
Emptiness is form.
-The Buddhist "Heart Scripture"

Tourette's Disease has a profound effect on the very personalities of those who suffer from it. Independent of the inherent changes the disease can make to the personality, it can also cause depression, withdrawal, denial, anger, and all sorts of other negative reactions. As we shall examine later, it could even be the cause of some commonly seen autistic symptoms. These reactions would be expected of, and found in, any individual ill or well, in the face of the kind of disability that TS creates. TS heaps upon the sufferer so many horrendous symptoms that seem bereft of meaning, empty; it is a miracle it does not cause total disintegration of the personality.

As a result, many patients are unwilling or unable to talk about their experiences with Tourette problems. Hopefully this book will speak for them, and I hope that they are not unhappy with what is said. The real dream I have for this book is that as you read it, you will hear the voices of all the unheard Tourette sufferers. "Form is emptiness, emptiness is form." Of course, all the opinions in this work, unless otherwise stated, are my own—garnered from many years' personal experience, study and research.

In memory and in the spirit of Joseph Bliss, the late TS patient who wrote such a fascinating account of the inner workings of TS, I offer a similar account. I will include a comprehensive bibliography of my favorite books and articles. In the past, many lay readers have been put off by the academic tone of what literature there is on the subject, something I wish to avoid as much as possible. (So please forgive the Preface!) This book will not duplicate Mr. Bliss' very clinical writing style. Instead, this work will endeavor to do two things as simply as possible from the vantage point of my personal experience: 1) Describe what it is really like to have Tourette Syndrome/autism; 2) Serve as an educational and perhaps diagnostic tool.

I hope to achieve these ends by sharing how Tourette Syndrome and autism shape every facet of life. Think of this not as an autobiography, but as the voice of Tourette Syndrome/autism. There is no comprehensive bibliography, because it would be longer than this book! But I think the bibliography I've cobbled together is as comprehensive as you could hope.

The emphasis will be slightly less in the direction of autism; I think more than enough autism books are gathering dust on shelves. Where I think it is most beneficial and useful, I will make mention of autism; you will have noted that I use the combined term "Tourette's Disease/autism" or else "TS/AS." I will repeat here that I believe that they are both manifestations of the same disease.

Shakespeare wrote, "There is a joy in being mad that only madmen know." It is emphatic that you know that TS/autistic patients are NOT mad; our joy is in being able to somehow educate others, to raise our voices, to understand ourselves, and to fight injustices however and whenever possible. For some of us, there is an obligation to fight in addition to the joy. There are so many for whom to fight, who cannot do anything about it and will never be able to do so.

We, as Tourette Disease sufferers and/or high function autism sufferers, must remember another Shakespeare quote: "…[W]hen the blast of war blows in our ears, then imitate the action of the tiger: summon up the blood, disguise fair nature with rage, and lend the eye a terrible aspect." Anon, my stalwart fellows, and let us lend the eye a terrible aspect, to remove the terrible aspect of the subject that is before us now! (That's the most Shakespearean prose you'll ever get out of me.)

Cry In The Wilderness: Tics

El sueño de la razón produce monstruos.
[When reason falls asleep, monsters are produced.]
-Francisco Goya, 18th century painter

I. What Tics Are

Imagine that you are sitting in a café with your family. At the table next to you is a handsome young man, perhaps twenty years old. He is tossing his head back and forth and making flailing motions with his elbow. He also rocks back and forth occasionally, causing his chair to creak loudly. Naturally you become distressed. He's also making odd hooting and whirring sounds. It is extremely uncomfortable, especially since your children are captivated by the sight of this young man. You may be asking yourself, "My God, look at that boy. Is he on drugs? Is he having a seizure? What will everyone think? What about the children?"

If only you could completely know his inner torment, and the iron discipline he invokes trying to fight what is happening to him. If only you could know all there is to know about this disease he is fighting. And you will know. Welcome to the world of Tourette Syndrome tics. A great deal has been written since the late 1980's about tics, probably the most prolific output since Dr. Tourette originally wrote about them. Tics: what you've just been seeing in your mind's eye, the gyrations and noises made by the boy at the café. There are a few excellent works dealing with tics, mainly magazine articles. Dr. Oliver Sacks has written some interesting items worth examining.

Dr. David Comings has written the definitive textbook on tics.

First we must have a good, clean definition in this matter. A tic is defined in Webster's College Dictionary as "a sudden, spasmodic, painless, involuntary muscular contraction, as of the face." *The Merck Manual* defines tics as "writhing, proximal postures." But actually, on the TS spectrum a tic is much more. There are vocal (phonic) tics: noises, voices, mimesis (what we simple lay people call mimicry, what I call "echophenomena"), repetition, speaking in accents; motor tics which can become very elaborate, involving any single part or combination of parts of the body including the parts no one can see; mental (what I call "internal") tics, those nasty buggers that seem to have much in common with obsessions; and finally emotional tics. A bit further on we will examine each kind of tic in turn.

I have recently read about "sensory" tics, and have no idea what these could be (perhaps tics of the senses, similar to perceptual disturbances). Let us define "tic" here as any involuntary behavior one could possibly imagine, and several unimaginable ones. Elaine Shimberg, author of *Living With Tourette Syndrome*, has coined the term "unvoluntary" to describe tics; she believes this new term is appropriate because tics are actually performed to relieve an inner compulsion. I don't see that as quite accurate, nor do I care much for this particular book. Tics are not voluntary, and you'll notice me reminding you of this every so often. Therefore I'll stick to "involuntary" because that is precisely what all tics are. Let's call a spade a spade!

Even in Samuel Johnson's day there was a fairly accurate conception of tics. But a century later, almost as soon as Dr. Tourette delineated their mechanism as best he could, he was ignored. Imagine it: in the 18th century, several of Johnson's friends proved by their actions and private writings that they had a clear grasp of the nature of his symptoms. They commended his courage in facing his disease.

This was mentioned contemporarily only to defend Johnson, because many others were expressing the opinion that his tics were simple neurosis or self-indulgence. Others, upon meeting him for the first time, thought he was severely retarded (an "ideot" [sic] as one fellow wrote). This erroneous opinion of tics persists to this very day. As we well know, a century after Dr. Johnson's friends defended him, Dr. Tourette wrote on the subject and he was ignored, and has been ignored ever since.

II: Chevreul Discovers the State of Mind of Involuntary Movement

In any discussion or exposition of neurological tics there should be some general discussion about involuntary movements. Would anyone be surprised to learn that there is commonly experienced involuntary movement in healthy people everyday? Well, if it does come as a surprise, this section is for you. Below we will explore fascinating research that dates back to the early 19th century, exposing and explaining the nature of a spectrum of involuntary muscular movement that is common to all animals, including humans.

It is a thrilling psychological as well as physiological exposé, and I believe it sheds much illumination on the nature of tics. Further, it not only clarifies the nature of what exactly we mean by "involuntary movement," but also presents some interesting points of view regarding the nature and origin of such movements in healthy people, who are totally unaffected by tics of any kind. It is an excellent préamble to a deeper study of tourettic tics.

Since the late 18th century (and undoubtedly for many centuries prior) there has been an obsession common in the West: the "magic pendulum" or "explorer's pendulum." This is nothing more than a plumb-bob hanging from a string or thread. The weight, when held, spins and oscillates "of its own accord"; they are often used to orient the occultist to a specific desired direction. Even today many dowsers use pointed plumb-bobs over maps, to locate water or missing people—the Nazis used the pendulums to predict American or ally attack locations. It is very much like the divining or dowser's rod. Today the pendulum is called the Chevreul Pendulum.

French chemist Michel-Eugène Chevreul (1786-1889) wrote an "open letter" in 1833 to the famous André Ampère, outlining his findings on the "explorer's/exploring pendulum." In brief, what Chevreul found was that it was his unconscious will that was creating involuntary movement in the hand holding the pendulum, thus causing the pendulum to swing. This dazzling find constitutes a vital component of involuntary movement research—and like his contemporaries Charcot, Itard, and de la Tourette, Chevreul is a forgotten figure. In his findings about involuntary movement and the pendulum that is now named after him, Chevreul laid some important psychomotor groundwork.

From time immemorial it has been recognized that the "magical" qualities of the pendulum appear only when it is hand-held. This had already led some scientists in the 18th century to conclude that the phenomenon must be "nervous," that is to say, nerve-related, in origin. Chevreul first studied the pendulum effect in 1812, though he did not publish the findings until much later, at Ampère's prompting. In 1853 the French Academy of Sciences appointed Chevreul chairman of a three-man committee that was to find and provide an answer to the mysterious pendulum effect.

The report, being the formal paper on the subject, was published in 1854. The title of this great work deserves to be spilled into our text in its glorious Gallic fullness, and is also cited in the bibliography under Tourette-related books: *"De la baguette divinatoire, du pendule dit explorateur et des tables tournantes, au point de vue de l'historie, de la critique et de la méthode éxperimentale"* ("Of the Divining Rod, the Explorer's Pendulum and Turning-Tables, From the Point of View of History, Critique, and the Experimental Method" [Paris: Mallet-Bachelier, 1854]). It gave the grand response to the riddle of the pendulum and other phenomena: it's all due to involuntary muscular movements caused by autosuggestion. In other words, the answer to the mystery is tics.

In 1852 the English physiologist William Carpenter had coined the term "ideo-motor" ("ideomotor") to describe these tics. It's a word that represents the fact that the idea, albeit unconscious, is what inspires the motor movements. This term astounds me even now—it's so close to my own term "echopersonae." According to Herman Spitz, the term "nicely encapsulates the fact that an involuntary motor response can be produced by a *dominant idea* [Italics mine]."

Sptiz, the author of the excellent "Skeptical Inquirer" article used for this section of the book, had become interested in Chevreul's work while examining claims about facilitated communication in 1997. Facilitated communication is the claim that autistic individuals who are not verbal can communicate either through a Ouija board, keyboard or label-printing machine. Of course, as Spitz and others have proved, "...the facilitators are unwittingly controlling [the autistic patient's] typing." This provides yet another link to my theory, and cannot be coincidental. But more on that later.

Spitz has written an excellent account of facilitated communication and other such phenomena in his 1997 book *Nonconscious Movements: From Mystical Messages to Facilitated Communication*. Into the general category of what I call the Chevreul Effect, Spitz includes table-turning (table-tilting), Ouija board movement, mind-reading, automatic handwriting and the "Clever Hans" Phenomenon. The "Clever Hans" Phenomenon, in which a horse-trainer, Willem von Osten, taught his horse Hans to answer simple mathematical problems by unconscious signals, should be called the "von

Osten Effect."

The "Clever Hans" Phenomenon is actually due to von Osten's involuntary movements, which trained the intelligent horse, rather than a reference to the horse's responses. Though it is true that audience response to the Clever Hans Phenomenon also falls into the category of the "Chevreul Effect," as they were insensible to von Osten's subtle tics, it is usually not considered as the primary area of interest. Anyway, when the great Chevreul died at the age of 102, on March 27, 1889, the funeral turnout was tremendous—thousands came to Notre Dame Cathedral to pay respects. But sadly, Chevreul was soon forgotten.

In the "Skeptical Inquirer" article, Spitz publishes for the first time the complete translation of Chevreul's "open letter" to Ampère; it is a thorough and fascinating work, worth quoting extensively. Chevreul begins by telling us exactly what he used for a pendulum in his experiments:

> *The pendulum I used was an iron ring hanging from a hemp thread; it had been put together by someone who keenly wished that I would verify for myself the phenomenon which took place when [the] person held [the pendulum] above water, a piece of metal, or a live being...*

Chevreul then explains how he held the pendulum, and suspended it in his right hand over a cistern of mercury, an anvil, and several animals. He wrote,

> *[If t]here were only a number of different bodies able to induce the pendulum's oscillations, it might be that by interpolating other bodies between these and the moving pendulum, it would come to a halt.*

How surprised he was when he saw that the interpolation of other objects decreased and finally stopped the oscillations. He noted that the oscillations resumed when the interfering bodies had been removed from between the pendulum and the experimental media. Chevreul wrote that "the more extraordinary those effects seemed to me, the more I felt the need to verify whether they were truly independent from any type of muscular movement in my arm...." Then he used a crutch to brace his arm while he held the pendulum; the closer the crutch got to his hand, the less movement there was in the pendulum. Finally it dawned on him:

> *[Using the crutch] caused me to think that quite probably a muscular movement that was taking place unbeknownst to me was determining the phenomenon, and I had to give even more consideration to this opinion, because I remembered, albeit vaguely, having been in quite a peculiar state... while my eyes were following the [pendulum's] oscillations.... I performed the experiment once again... [and] I was feeling very clearly that at the same time as my eyes were following the oscillating pendulum, there was in myself a disposition or tendency toward movement, which, as involuntary as it seemed to me, was proportionately more satisfied as the pendulum [moved more]....*

It occurred to Chevreul that because of the nature of this monumental discovery, he might be able to prove it conclusively by blindfolding himself. This he ordered to be done while he was holding the magic pendulum, which was swinging in wide arcs at the time. The instant he was blindfolded, his involuntary movement stopped, and so did the pendulum. Then, still blindfolded, Chevreul had his assistant place and remove interfering bodies between the pendulum and the experimental media. The pendulum remained totally still for fifteen solid minutes. Thus Chevreul came up with a complete interpretation for the phenomenon:

> *While I was holding the pendulum in my hand, a muscular movement in my arm, though unfelt by me, made the pendulum [move], and the oscillations, once begun, were soon augmented by the influence which sight exerted to put me into that peculiar state of disposition or tendency toward movement... this muscular movement, albeit increased by this very same disposition, is... weak enough to come to a stop... as soon as one merely has the thought of trying to determine whether some given thing will stop it. Hence there is an intimate relationship... between the execution of certain movements and the action of the thought relative to them, though that thought is not yet a deliberate will commanding the [muscles].*

Chevreul was so impressed and humbled by his findings that he repeatedly and in vain tried to reproduce the pendulum's oscillations—then further discovered that because he knew the reason for the movements, *the pendulum would not oscillate in his hand at all.*

He seemed to have caught on by noting that in the original experiment, the interpolation of foreign bodies stopped the movement— since he did sort of expect such an action to stop it. He then goes on to explain his two main facts: that the pendulum can move without the holder's knowledge of what causes it, and that as the holder watches it move, he unconsciously causes it to move more. Thus the stopping of the pendulum during the interpolation of a separate object only intensified the movement once movement resumed, after the interfering body was removed.

He brilliantly cites the example of the dowsing or divining rod. Chevreul believed that, if the dowser is not blindfolded and can see the terrain, he will unconsciously recognize a place most likely to hide water, and that the diviner will involuntarily move his rod toward that place. The closer he gets to that place and the more he recognizes the signs of water there—such as green grass and lush vegetation—the more strongly he and his dowsing rod will move toward that place, involuntarily.

Chevreul goes on to list a number of instances in which this very phenomenon takes place, though we of course cannot really be aware of it at the time it occurs. In fact we are never aware of it. He mentions watching a bird in flight, or a stone being thrown, and the body's tendency to follow the movement; he also mentions how a bowler or pool-player follows the ball with his body, in essence trying to "will" the ball to go where desired. Chevreul was astonished to realize that one's tendency to move in this way is unaffected even by the physical impossibility of moving. He illustrates further:

> *I believe that in ordinary falls [as in a person falling down], letting fall [as in allowing oneself to fall] causes less inconvenience than the effort made to prevent the fall. It is in that sense that I understand the truth of the proverb: There is a god [sic] for children and for drunkards.*

Chevreul then cites instances such as a person being on a cliff, or on a narrow suspended bridge over a great height. He notes that the person, out of fear, unwillingly throws his body in the direction opposite from where he thinks danger lies. Conversely, Chevreul notes the simultaneous tendency to be "frozen" in fear. After this, Chevreul leads us into new territory that may have enormous importance to the echophenomenal tics found in Tourette's Disease and autism:

> *The tendency to [move] in a specific direction, resulting from the attention given to a certain object, seems to me the primary cause of several phenomena usually attributed to imitation... [such as] yawning [and] the communicability of laughter... There is no doubt in my mind that the sight of certain specific actions strongly influence our frail machinery, that a narrative of such actions [vocal and motor], or... even... the knowledge one acquires of [these actions] through mere reading, incline certain individuals toward those same actions, thus following a tendency to [move in a way] that [the person] never would have thought... an action to which they would never have been driven by what one must call instinct....*

So, we see that Chevreul has actually delineated two very normal conditions, not one: autosuggested tics, and other-suggested (what I like to call "exosuggested") tics. Spitz calls them "nonconscious" movements, but I feel this may be an inaccurate if not slightly misleading definiens. I insist this, because we are dealing with none other than involuntary movement, the same as the tics we see in Tourette and autistic symptomology. To call them "nonconscious" suggests to me a sort of deliberate but blocked state of mind—and that is certainly not the case. In proof of my view, Chevreul ingeniously notes that a certain "state" is required to cause these phenomena of involuntary, self-caused (autosuggested) or echophenomenal (exosuggested) tics.

We know that there is no known "state of mind" other than disease which causes tics in Tourette Disease and autism. When the healthy person is not in Chevreul's "state of susceptibility," Chevreul gleefully notes, that person will not experience these involuntary movements. In his emphasis on a "state," Chevreul gives the lie to Spitz's descriptor "nonconscious"—the state may be nonconscious, yes, but not the tics. The tics are totally involuntary, completely unconscious. Chevreul in fact puts great emphasis on this "state," which is none other than a certain state of mind, and closes his paper with an explanation of just what this state of mind can do:

> *There is nothing more curious [in the sphere of human action]...than the knowledge of the means used by the salesman to... first attract and then fix the buyer's attention on the qualities of the object which he wants him to purchase, nothing more curious than the knowledge of the means used by the conjurer... to make [a person] pick one card rather than another from the deck, or to [distract the*

> *spectator]... The outcome of these considerations is that completely different trades use... similar means [:] that of securing man's attention, in order to later exert a specific effect on him.*

Chevreul seems very much like Tourette, deeply interested in mimesis and echophenomena. It's pretty clear that Chevreul has outlined a natural, healthy form of tic, shared by all animals including humans. The final blow comes when Chevreul again emphasizes that many animals, in fact, experience this kind of involuntary thought and movement—not animal instinct, he says, but the very same phenomena that occur with us. Though this remark of Chevreul's evokes shades of Grandin's cows, I have difficulty determining what animal "instincts" Chevreul might be referring to—and he himself sheds no further light on it. Perhaps he is referring to the charming of snakes, the training of animals á là Clever Hans, or the behaviors that animals learn from their own species. Perhaps he refers to things that animals are able to learn from humans.

The final paragraph of Chevreul's paper reminds us that knowledge of man comes from the study of animals and animal faculties; he insists that "before attempting to compose a general system of philosophy, it is necessary to have collected as vast a number as possible of groups of analogous facts, and moreover the facts in each group must have been previously investigated in depth..." Amen, Docteur Chevreul!

There is an interesting pair of events Chevreul emphasizes, which I believe connects his observations to TS and Asperger's autism. He mentions a "state" and a simultaneous inclination toward movement that ultimately results in movement. Both, which Chevreul seems to separate into two distinct events, are involuntary and unconscious. It seems that the "state" could be related to autism, and the movements could be related to Tourette movements. In other words, Chevreul's effect is on the healthy, normal end of the spectrum, and neurological psychomotor diseases are on the other end. The fact that the "state" of mind and the movement can be separated into distinct events, as autism and Tourette Disease are distinct diseases, gives credence to my theory.

Chevreul himself supports this when he observes that as soon as the "state" is eradicated, the tics are gone forever. What we will continue groping to understand is the distinction between the known stimulus of Chevreul (the "state" that can be understood, thus eradicated) and the unknown stimulus of Tourette/autism. But I am confident that the stimuli involved in Chevreul Effects and in diseases are of the same type. Remember, Chevreul's experiments and observations are of the normal, healthy human responses. What might those responses be if we examined neurologically disabled people?

In the next section we will be able to compare tic manifestation with Chevreul's studies of healthy involuntary movement, as we were able to compare Chevreul with the history of tic diseases. There is a mysterious connection that is hard to make out—a link hinted at in Chevreul's work that finds its fruition in de la Tourette's work.

Perhaps in looking at and understanding tics—as we now understand involuntary movement disease research history and healthy involuntary movement—we will arrive at an answer to this particular mystery. Just as Chevreul and de la Tourette answered other mysteries so long ago....

III. How Tics Manifest

...[B]ad habit, my dear. Do you guard against bad habits?

-Dr. Samuel Johnson, explaining his tics to a little girl who asked about them

Chevreul was on to something big. With his research in mind, we can proceed to study Tourettic involuntary movements, which have borne so many labels over the centuries. Tics seem to begin as incredible "urges," wrongly compared to the urge to sneeze. The urge to tic has a classification all its own. It's a combination of the "urge" to sneeze, the "need" to do something to feel better, and the Parkinson patient's "desire" to tremble—none of which have anything directly to do with voluntary urges or desires at all, as the great Chevreul's work implies.

As far as I can tell, sometimes it seems I am compelled to tic simply because I know I have TS. Or as a friend once observed, "You're doing it because now, you know you have to." But the "urge" and its ultimate "relief," which is the tic itself, are both really one mechanism working in tandem. It is one seamless, progressive action if you like, and utterly involuntary.

I recently watched a documentary showing a Tourette patient being placed into an MRI. Electrodes were wired to the patient's face, in order to record brain activity and tics simultaneously. What was discovered was that the movement, like all movement, begins in the reptilian part of the brain. But rather than passing through to the "movement-willing" and "judgement" centers, which is normal, the signal simply moves to the nerves themselves. Thus, many Tourette sufferers describe an "urge" which finds "satisfaction" in the tics. What we are really feeling is that the brain is up to something—we know not what—and before we know it, the whole process has resulted in a tic.

Later we might say it seemed like an urge—a formless "golem"—that was finally given the form of a tic. When the same test was performed on a healthy person who was asked to mimic the tics, an expected and typical pattern of brain activity was clearly evident. In other words, where the healthy control showed a typical pattern of willing the action, thinking it through, and then performing it, the TS patient showed none of this brain pattern activity. The "order to move" was simply "given" in the reptilian part of the brain, then immediately executed. It's the Chevreul Effect gone haywire, coming out of nowhere.

Thus even before we start, we've already encountered the potential for a dizzying array of possible tics. Even the Chevreul Effect can be fairly said to be tic activity in healthy people, albeit stimulated by something external. Perhaps tics in Tourette Disease and autism are stimulated in this way—but if so, the external cause is invisible to us, yet to be discovered. As it stands we know that tics are internally stimulated, as if by electrode, such as the electrode-stimulated movement we might see in evoked response tests. If only Chevreul and Tourette had worked together!

So I am very anxious to be as exact as possible in my comments and descriptions. In this book you will find I have coined a number of terms which previously had no name. I would like to pause here to offer such a term: palipraxia. This is physical self-mimicry. Professionals might think of it as simply a tic of repetition, a manifestation of compulsive behavior, or autistic self-stimulation. I can assure you that none of these is really the case.

Palipraxia relates to the self as echopraxia (mimicking the movements of others) relates to others, yet it has never been discussed. I'll give you two good examples: sometimes when I scratch my head, I may notice my reflection in the window or someplace. I then mimic my own actions. It is done in the same way we tend to mimic others: I'm done with scratching my head, but now I experience a tic that causes me to mimic myself, and has nothing to do with scratching at all.

Also, I tend to repeat things I've said in the past, mimicking myself or simply verbalizing the words all over again. The experts do have a name for this activity: palilalia. This seems to be a special class of tic behavior: not easy to describe, not easy to live with, because others tend to view it as being deliberately irritating or facetious. It probably isn't a very common tic, either—though I've noticed that a number of my family members do it.

I have personally observed that these particular tics tend to be either lifelong or very short-lived. Other tics are generally somewhere in between these extremes. Perhaps Chevreul was close to discovering something like this; there is something behind this tic activity that might teach us more in the future, as Tourette himself noted.

It is true, as Dr. Sacks pointed out in his revised notes to "A Surgeon's Life," that everyday events, activities, people's names, or sounds can become "enshrined" in vocal and motor tics. Some patients, according to him, report that their tics are almost a sort of life archive. This I find to be true for me. These kinds of tics are a remembrance, an involuntary mental monument of something that made an extremely strong impression. Perhaps something like a song one hears so often that it reverberates in the memory for years, causing memories and emotional reactions. For instance, I had very bad balance as a child and became accustomed to grasping anything nearby for support. Ever since then, when I become upset, I reach out in a lunge to grab something that isn't there.

This lunging behavior is a good example of a common tic, which is generally described as "throwing out" or "flailing" the hands and arms. Tics can last at the very most a few months, though some simple ones can be lifelong. My best friend of two decades is nicknamed "Boo," and a frequent tic I experience during elation is a set of variations on that word. I start with "boo," progressing to "boodly-boo," and so on, until I'm spent! I've had this tic for at least seven years running. A tic that goes back to my childhood, the oldest one, is my eye-squeezing; the second oldest tic I have is adjusting my glasses. And these are just the tics I am aware of—I know there are others of which I have always been unaware. This is common.

A very embarrassing period was the "kitty, kitty, kitty!" tic: I used to call my favorite cat this way, in a silly high-pitched voice, as do most people. I began doing that whenever I spotted someone I knew. Lucky me: they all had a good sense of humor. At least I didn't snap my fingers and whistle at them! Oddly enough, I never developed this tic with my previous cats, nor did it reoccur with my later cats, after my darling little kitty passed away. I also commonly express thoughts with complex movements, sound effects, bizarre jokes or voices. All these are tic activity, and yet it seems I can almost feel myself "choosing" to do these things.

Undoubtedly that is a "lizard brain" sensation, the feeling of having somehow willed what is unwilled. This is why Elaine Shimberg calls tics "unvoluntary," much the way Spitz refers to the tics of a healthy person as "nonconscious," but they are not "unvoluntary" nor are they "nonconscious." One may choose to varying degrees how to express one's propensities, but one's propensities are genetically preordained (non-determinists be damned!). We can most certainly NOT choose exactly how to manifest the symptoms of a disease—any disease. As Schopenhauer wrote, we can do whatever we want but cannot will what we want. The reptilian part of the brain should be a reminder of that.

Nor is this to say that tics are a mode of expression. Far from it! We may say, to add support to the previous paragraph, that tics can sometimes accompany our normal expressions in a predictable way. Yet they are not expressions of anything *pro se* other than purely physical symptoms. We can see how Dr. Tourette could have made the mistake of assuming that motor tics are always simultaneously accompanied by vocal ones, wondering if the motor action forces a vocal action or if the same stimulus forces both actions simultaneously. TS patients do sometimes use these "tourettisms" (to borrow Dr. Sacks' term) as a coping mechanism to handle the intense strain of the illness.

Dr. Sacks has concluded, rather accurately I think, that many neurologically ill people find ways of employing their symptoms in a subtly and harmlessly "manipulative" way. I've done it myself, mostly to impress other people with the TS, in a sense "manipulating" them into seeing and accepting it. Still, tics are not a pretty sight. A few of the tics I've described thus far are vocal, and of a specific kind, which I call "seman-tics." My above examples are but a fragment; I'll return to explain the topic of "seman-tics" later.

Motor tics are a little different in nature than vocal ones. When I was still a Catholic, I received many dirty looks for the head-toss that always appeared during Mass. My family almost broke my arms for my infamous hand-flapping, which they thought was too feminine for a boy. I was almost escorted from the mall for the shoulder-shrug-elbow-jerk that nearly took out a little old lady's eye. I was almost kicked out of grade school because I couldn't sit still or stop talking in weird voices. Then there was the really disastrous period. My parents often came dangerously close to selling me on the black market: I needed too many wardrobe and eyeglasses replacements. Everything kept getting mysteriously destroyed, by me in the throes of terrible motor tics.

After having learned of Chevreul's studies, imagine experiencing such involuntary movements all the time, with no apparent or logical reason. Think of the stimulus snowballing inside you. Imagine the feeling of having this movement build in the brain, without knowing what's going on, and suddenly experiencing the final outcome: an embarrassing tic.

Years later I would never forgive a co-worker, who after witnessing a series of tics, even though I had explained TS to her, asked me why I was so "stupid" and did such "stupid things." This she loudly asked in front of more than two dozen people in the middle of the county court house. I wheeled on her and replied, "I don't know why, this is a disease I have. Why do you ask such stupid questions?" Would you like to know why we TS patients are so "stupid"?

Imagine you are in the hands of a mad doctor. He is experimenting with sending electrical signals to the brain, and has you hooked up like a Christmas tree to hundreds of implanted, remote controlled electrodes. He sends you on your way, free as a bird. Yet all he has to do is punch his keypad, and he can enjoy watching you twirl, ballet-style. Or maybe he makes you jump before you enter a doorway. Perhaps he causes you to roll or dart your eyes, especially while driving (this eye movement is called "oculogyric crisis").

The good doctor may be in a mood to really amuse himself, so he makes you pump your hips at passersby. (I know, I know. Many doctors are idiots and couldn't even imagine all this.) In spite of our sometimes whimsical coping methods, this is the truth about tics. Most of the time it's even worse, and there is no evil "Dr. Mengele" to blame. We don't even have the benefit of the Chevreul Effect, the "ideomotorisms," to explain the tics away.

Many severe TS patients are in perpetual motion (not me, I'm a "moderately severe" case but exercise a frightening control, which I learned through Buddhism). A good instance is someone like the great lexicographer Dr. Samuel Johnson. He was always rocking and rolling, jerking, bobbing and weaving, hopping and stamping. His friend and biographer John Boswell gives many examples in his Life of Samuel Johnson, and there are some other Johnson biographies that describe his tics and OCD at some length. As I mentioned, his tics were so severe that many upon meeting him for the first time assumed that Dr. Johnson was retarded.

Naturally, Johnson was a target: a famous comedian, somewhat like a stand-up performer, was famous for doing impressions. David Garrett was his name, and he was actually fond of Johnson. But he went too far imitating the poor doctor's most vulnerable and helpless moments. When Dr. Johnson heard about Garrett's comedy routine, he had word sent to Garrett that he was going out to buy a "double length" oak staff. Dr. Johnson said he would visit Garret and take his new staff with him, to see how well Garrett could imitate him then. Garrett got the message and ceased; after all, Johnson was a very powerful, athletic man in spite of his girth.

For those TS patients who tic violently and constantly, a very tough life is always going to be the result. Some remain housebound. Others go on bravely with life, and some have become famous. Later we will read about Thelonious Monk, the legendary jazz composer and pianist who ticced his way through a life that was already terrible to begin with.

Before moving on, I want to address an interesting motor tic: I call it the "touching tic." I cannot seem to find the formal term for it anywhere in my research, so I offer a new and improved term: tactipraxia, literally, "touching movement." It involves touching the self, other people and/or objects, using various parts of the body, especially the hands. I'm certain that a similar term, copropraxia, exists in the literature to denote any kind of obscene touching or gestures.

When I think of the touching tic, which has featured strongly in my life though not in any obscene manifestation, I tend to lump together all the tics that I think fall into this category: licking the self or others, biting or touching things with the teeth, lips, or tongue, grabbing, holding, hitting, caressing or fondling the self or others, and any kind of inappropriate or obscene touching. It isn't clear to me if the sniffing tic fits in this group. (Quite a bit of the source literature describing these types of motor tics exists thanks to Dr. David Comings.) If it sounds alarming, believe me, it is. Much more so to the TS patient than anyone.

Tactipraxia is an embarrassing subgroup of symptoms, so people tend to run away or make a big production of tic behavior in general. It is wise to do neither of these. Acceptance and humor are the best remedies; simply ignoring tics is a big favor that people can do for us. Often the touching can involve one's own genitals or the genitals of others; I knew a kid who touched his and others' chests; you can imagine the nightmare that such a symptom can cause.

A TS patient who suffers with this particular symptom, as well as friends and loved ones, should never ignore it. Pertinent to this touching symptom, there is a clip of Mahmoud Abdoul-Rauf (Chris Jackson) of the Denver Nuggets basketball team. The clip is in Laurel Chiten's documentary "Twist and Shout." It shows a basketball game in progress; an opposing player is crossing Mahmoud's path. Mahmoud suddenly reaches out and gingerly "fondles" the player's waist. You can see the eye-popped astonishment on the player's face as he mumbles, "What... what're you doin'?"

To which Mahmoud smoothly replies, "Just givin' you a little backrub, man." It is rather comical, but the humiliated expression on Mahmoud's face is painfully apparent.

When something like this happens, explaining it to others is not a bad idea. When we are embarrassed and try to behave nonchalantly, people definitely get the impression that we're trying to get away with something. Many TS sufferers avoid being in public if they absolutely can do nothing to control touching tics. When I'm in public, I try to substitute these types of tics with others—but then, I don't really like touching or being touched, and that serves as a strong deterrent. We will deal with the concept of tic substitution shortly.

The Ella Fitzgerald Tendency: Vocal Tics

When I've reflected on vocal tics, it has occurred to me that society is always very annoyed with individuals who make noises of any kind. You just can't imagine the red-faced tizzy I experience after a day of people giving me mean looks because I've been too noisy. Vocal tics can consist of any noise; many of these noises lean toward the comical or disturbing. Often, vocal tics can take a form such as the "scat" singing style of Ella Fitzgerald, Scatman Cruthers or Cab Calloway. But such things as "barnyard" noises, mechanical noises, cartoon voices, or foreign accents are the commonest vocal tics, all of which I suffer daily.

Now, I do try having fun with these tics as often as possible, and this is useful, bearing in mind that TS patients become masters of tic camouflage. As an instance, when I'm in a car with others and I make noises, I try to be very covert. The whole way, everyone is asking, "Do you hear that? What is wrong with the car? Is it the car? What could that BE?" It's a real hoot. Then when I'm found out (IF I'm found out), everyone has a good laugh about it. Most of the time, I go into fits of laughter once I get away from the people and can see that they are just as disturbed by the sudden cessation of the noise.

Vocal tics are never really fun, though. They are disruptive in much the same way as motor tics. Among the simple tics, there is loud inhaling or exhaling, stuttering, repeating words two or three times, speaking with no control over pitch, volume, speed or modulation. We see these exact tics in autism. Then there is what is called "blocking," when the speaker is stopped cold every few words or sentences. This is not the same as aphasia, which is the inability to recollect a particular word; aphasia is mostly seen in stroke patients.

For a few seconds, the rest of a sentence just doesn't seem to want to issue forth. (I call this symptom "sticking," and I have "sticking" motor tics too, in which I freeze momentarily. As we shall see later, this "freezing" is seen in autism as well.) These vocalic stopping or stalling tics especially seem to manifest simultaneously with motor tics; perhaps this is the reason Dr. Tourette thought motor and vocal tics accompanied each other all the time. Then the tics progress to any and every imaginable noise, right up to actual shrieking. Like the motor tics, vocal/phonic tics can consist of anything that involves the throat, larynx, mouth, and/or nose.

We then have more complex types of vocal tics: all types of mimicry, impressions, accents, "weird" speech patterns, and all varieties of sound effects. This category also includes "natural" sounds such as throat-clearing (a common one), hawking, coughing or rasping. Snorting and sniffling, however, seem to fall into the motor tic category, as does throat clicking (or "clucking"), which has lead some doctors to misdiagnose respiratory or allergy troubles. It's interesting to note how the motor and vocal tics can seem to blend into one another.

My father, for example, has a tic that progresses something like this: "hmm-sniff-grunt-snort-cough-bark." It sounds like a Great Dane choking on grass. He does this tic about every three minutes, and has been suffering from the tic all his life. The rest of the family, to my utter amazement, has the same tic. It's less frequent but when anyone does it, they sound exactly like my father. One day during a family gathering, one of my brothers was coming up the walk. My father was inside, just having finished talking to one of my sisters. My brother did "Dad's Tic," and my sister was startled. She said, "How the hell did dad get outside so fast?" As is typical, none of them realize that they have this tic. Another tic my father has which we all suffer is a sort of "roaring-lion" throat-clearing. Again, very typical in the realm of vocal tics, and typically unrecognized by the family.

That particular tic is actually famous: it's the infamous old Jewish man hacking, a favorite character of comedian Billy Crystal. He has been quoted as saying that not only did his uncle do the noise, but "most old Jewish men

I saw [when I was] growing up." It has struck me that whenever a comedian or movie star performs the character of an old Jewish man, they always add this particular tic. Whether it's racism or just a gross sense of humor, I don't know. Coming from a Sephardic Jewish family, I can say that almost every male in our entire family does have that tic.

For a while, the TS scholars were trying to decide how to classify, say, throat noises that vocalize and other nasopharyngeal noises that don't vocalize. A few paragraphs ago we looked at this question. Well, it turns out that our answer is right under our noses: if the tic actually vocalizes, it's a vocal tic. Anything else, even if it makes a noise, is a motor tic. A good example is my father's "lion roar," or a strong exhaling, which is a common tic. If it is produced with a noise (like "AHHHHHHHH!") then it's a vocal tic. If it's just blowing wind like a whale, no matter how hard, it's motor. But many experts still classify vocal tics as any tic of the nasopharyngeal-oral apparatus. This blurry line is what fascinated Dr. Tourette so much that he thought vocal and motor tics had to go hand-in-hand.

Finally in the vocal tic category there is the fixation with words or sounds themselves, and even fixation with silence. I believe this "fixation" is the root of vocal tics, and it is no coincidence that we find this same symptom in autism. Dr. Sacks writes of his patient, Dr. Morton Duran of Canada, whose children kept a list of favorite words; Dr. Duran called them "candy for the mind." He enjoyed verbalizing these words, and they helped take the place of his more annoying vocal tics. I find there is an interesting correlation between such word tics and the non-stop, pedagogic "lecturing" seen in Asperger's Autism (what is commonly called the "Little Professor" feature). Later you will read examples of these kinds of tics.

Seman-tics

As a small child, not yet in kindergarten, I had invented a complete and complex language of words and sounds for everything that had meaning for me. I must have sounded like a little Martian. I did not know that this was a good way to express vocal tics. I've also learned that this is extremely common to high functioning autistic children, especially those with deficiencies in comprehension. I'm not really so sure I can find a proper description for it. It is truly as close to involuntary, I would even say reflexive, as one can get. I perceive it is a more reflexive type activity than other tics, or perhaps it is a way of filtering out the confusing sensory input.

Perhaps in considering this manifestation we are actually in the waters of autism. The 'seman-tics' surely evolve from this symptom, be it an autistic or Tourettic symptom: viz., I had no real comprehension of the proper word for something, but I had my own word for it, or at least a sound effect that indicated it. Often I found myself in the pit of despair, enunciating the word or making the sound over and over again, while the adults around me floundered in confusion.

When I watched "A Rage for Order," Dr. Sacks' fabulous documentary about Jessy Parks, the autistic artist, I was reminded of my semantics when her family talked about the word "gake." Jessy had first written the word to describe something—her parents were unsure of what the meaning was. Her parents did not even know Jessy was capable of understanding letters. Much later they realized that "gake" was Jessy's onomatopoeic rendition of the sounds made by the old radiators in the house; "gake" simultaneously represented Jessy's perception of, interest in, and fear of the radiator, ultimately revealing her fear of the furnace in the basement and the particularly loud radiator in her parents' bedroom. At the same time the "gake" was a calling of attention to her hypersensitive hearing.

At present, I don't invent too many new words—but as you've read this book you must have noted my delight in inventing "correct" new terms for symptoms. As a child, almost half the things I recognized continued to bear names I had given them. It was some time before I became aware of their proper names. In looking back I notice that seman-tics is not baby talk, but something resembling actual words in another language. Many of the words I used were onomatopoeic, and this may have been an indication of attempting to decipher the world, as Jessy Parks does.

Still, I had no trouble communicating verbally with others if I wanted, though there were periods when I lapsed into a mysterious autistic silence. I've read that HF autistic people risk a spiraling descent into more severe autism during emotional upheavals, and I think that's what my silences are. During stress or upset, people who suffer Tourette's Disease and Asperger's Autism plunge deeply into a loss of control, becoming totally disabled by a multitude of symptoms. It's almost like an instant multiple sclerosis.

One of my most common vocal tics, which I've suffered all my life, is talking to myself aloud. I not only talk; I have discussions, arguments, do my version of commercials, and even give lectures! It is still not clear to me why this happens. It seems I can't think properly unless I talk to myself, think aloud as it were. It annoys me to no end. Mostly I do this when alone. I learned long ago not to do this in front of anyone. Though I do get caught by other drivers talking to myself in my car, I pretend I'm talking into a recorder or singing to myself. It has been recently indicated that this is also a very common feature of HF autistic people; some think that autistic people help themselves understand and remember by talking to themselves in this way.

The great inventor Nikola Tesla (and Samuel Johnson) had the talking-aloud tic among other symptoms (as did Tesla's father, according to Tesla's autobiography). No one has come forward to declare whether Tesla suffered from Tourette Syndrome or autism, but I think he suffered from both conditions. He is famous for his monstrous case of OCBs. In any case, it is not necessary to go into any examples of the trouble talking to yourself can cause; I leave it to your imagination, and your imagination will not fail you.

Another frequent symptom of mine (again found in all HF autistics) was my tendency to perform 'commercials', which were always fun. As a kid I tended to mimic entire television and radio commercials. I enjoyed inventing my own two-minute spots; my parents thought I would be a TV announcer or one hell of a salesman. I was using these to communicate with myself and others. If there was a question of going someplace to eat, for example, my preference was indicated by doing the appropriate commercial. It was a part of my learning experience—that is unless I altered my version of the commercial with, shall we say, blue language.

When I found something to my extreme liking, I made up a "television commercial" or jingle to indicate it. Even though this tendency may not exactly fit as a complex phonic tic, you will notice that the more interesting tics tend to be vocal ones. The complex motor tics tend to limit themselves to stereotyped movements, gestures, dance-like positions and physical mimesis. These commercial spots I performed as a child have ultimately resulted in my not being able to tolerate hearing even a few seconds of any commercial. Thank God for the mute button! Now if only I had one of those on myself....

The seman-tics are really quite interesting. It seems that certain words, whether part of real or invented language, can stick in the brain much like a perfect image of the newspaper sticks to Silly Putty. Now, if the words are imposed upon the brain in this fashion, they must be spoken. To a degree it is a matter of sensuality: it feels delicious to say them. For me, it can come close to a sexual experience. The feel of the vocal cords working, the tongue, lips and teeth in concert, is almost as good as sex! The tic is final release and sometimes I can't stop until I'm exhausted, no matter what type of tics I'm having. Their expression is basically like a "neurological orgasm." Dr. Duran's list of words, his "candy for the mind," reflect this comparison beautifully.

Again, it is the underlying involuntary neurological urge needing expression and satisfaction that causes tics to erupt. This word or image-sticking is an excellent example of the "life archiving" that Dr. Sacks mentioned. The same is true of speaking in weird or foreign accents. As a teen, I always had lots of fun calling a store and asking about products of interest in a Bengali accent. But don't get the idea that this is mischief, though we TS patients are prone to it. Always remember: we really can't help it.

Echopersonae: Being Another To Be Oneself

Doing voices is something of a separate tic activity, mimicry. It can generally be termed mimesis, but I prefer to call it echopersonae, because there is a spectrum and at the far end we find a total mimicry that is hard to define because it runs so deeply. We are in an area where imitative vocal and motor tics can blend, and in the case of echopersonae, they take the entire personality, the entire psyche, with them.

This assimilation of anything from an accent or vocal inflection to a whole personality is considered by many doctors to be the extreme form of echopraxia, physical mimesis. In his excellent book on Asperger's Autism, Tony Attwood reveals that echopersonae (he does not use my term—he uses the older expression "take off") is common in Asperger sufferers. He feels that in such cases the echopersonae helps the socially inept sufferer learn how to speak and act properly.

"Echopersonae" involves a lot of echolalia. The fact is, my experience is that this is a separate tic that is a deeply complex, symbiotic combination of echopraxia and echolalia. (Thus the official term, echophenomena.) In the future echophenomena will probably be a major branch of TS study, and it is a good term to describe any echo-tic that does not involve "echopersonae," though for that purpose I like "echo-tic." In the next section you will read how any echo-tic could, on the other hand, be a form of obsession, and you should bear in mind that this array of tic activity is really very common in the autistic spectrum. Still, I am like Dr. Tourette, who was most fascinated by this aspect relative to TS.

In echopersonae, the extreme manifestation is the assimilation of someone's character and surface personality in toto. Normally this doesn't last long, and I believe that in this extreme form it is very rare (though as I said above, Tony Attwood found it to be almost universal among Asperger's Autism patients). As I say, I think the term echopersonae is very accurate for this set of tics because it can become so complete—it actually becomes a *persona*, which in the plural is *personae*.

As an example, I am a big fan of Peter Falk's Lieutenant Columbo character. When the series began airing, I became Columbo. It wasn't fanaticism or psychosis. It just happened: the gravelly voice, the rumpled raincoat (yes, I owned one), the cigar that was always unlit, the messy hair, the absentmindedness. I echopersonaed the whole character. Why I needed to echo the entire character is a mystery; probably it was due to some childhood strains long forgotten.

Then one day, Columbo was gone from me. My mother complains that my Columbo period ruined my posture (he had a slouch, remember?). On the upside, it added to my strengths, as all instances of echopersonae do. Even one of my attorneys once complemented me, saying, "You're better than Columbo." Dr. Oliver Sacks is to be thanked for first mentioning the extreme echo-tics in his book *The Man Who Mistook His Wife for a Hat,* in the chapter entitled "The Possessed." Dr. Sacks mentions echopersonae (again, not using my term) manifesting in sufferers of what he calls "Super Tourette's."

Sacks wondered if such severe assimilation of another's personality or characteristics could cause a disintegration of the personality. I heartily disagree that this could be the case. Dr. Sacks feels that such a symptom is "a tic of the whole personality," and that is an assertion I can accept. However, if echopersonae is a sustained, ultra-complicated tic, as Sacks and I both believe, then it casts new light on the nature, duration and detail of all tics, whether Tourettic or autistic. Finally, I cannot agree with Sacks line of questioning the disintegration of the patient's personality because as I stated, echopersonae is a process, and it ultimately comes to an end. When it does, the sufferer comes out of it for the better.

Personally I don't think that any of the echo-tics are too difficult to understand. Didn't you like to pretend you were a monkey, ghost or windstorm when you were a kid? Didn't you sometimes try to dress and act like mom or dad, even borrowing their clothes? As a child, the whole nature and life of another being or phenomenon is absorbed; during play, we imagine how a gust of wind "thinks"; we imagine how a monkey reasons; we imagine what a ghost might "like to eat." Then we act these things out, but they grow from sharp observation. Echo-tics are like that.

On the other side of the coin, as I mentioned, echopersonae might be a bit like when you wished you could be just like dad in every way, so you tried to "become" him, talking and acting like him, perhaps even borrowing his clothes, sneaking a few pats of his after-shave or even shaving with his razor. Of course with autism, echo-tics are called "parroting" and "mimicry," since doctors think of autistics as mindless creatures. I believe autism demonstrates the same principal as TS when it comes to mimesis or echopersonae. In any case we do see quite a bit of echoing and mimicking in healthy children of all ages; perhaps, as is so often the case, we are looking at something completely normal that is blasted out of proportion by disease.

The Devil At Every Turn: "Demonic Possession" and Tourette Disease

In the 1940s a teenager in St. Louis, Missouri, began to suffer a buildup of Tourette symptoms. These had been triggered by the death of his beloved aunt, who was involved in the occult. The symptoms culminated in extreme echopersonae of religious figures, chiefly Satan and the Archangel Michael, along with a wide range of other tics. When motor tics manifested and things began flying about the house at blinding speed, and when the voices grew weirder and more violent, the situation became so nerve-wracking that the boy's parents believed he was possessed by the devil.

The boy's case is unusual since he'd had no noticeable symptoms before, and apparently the symptoms eventually vanished. Before any improvements were to be seen, a Roman Catholic exorcism was recommended to the Protestant parents by their own minister. The exorcism, once approved, lasted almost a year, culminating at a mental hospital run by the famous medical Alexian Order of monks. It is notable that only after the involvement of the Church did the boy began to echolate religious figures. Decades later, author William Blatty got his hands on the diary which had been kept by one of the Alexian brothers who had cared for the boy during the final major exorcism.

The legend holds that the room where "Satan left the boy once and for all" was immediately sealed, never to be opened again. During demolition of the old hospital in the 1970's, someone happened to rummage through the desk in the room. A copy of the legendary but never before seen diary had been found in the top drawer! Blatty used this case history as the basis for his novel, *The Exorcist*. Of course, the boy's true identity and present whereabouts are kept in absolute secrecy, though a young seminarian involved in the exorcism as an assistant, who is today an active parish priest, has given interviews about general facts of this case. He has conveyed that the boy grew up to be a fine, healthy man with a couple of children and a good family life.

It is possible that the boy, who is listed in the secret diary as "Robby," may have suffered from a viral infection of some sort, a scenario that is now known to cause sudden but temporary tourettic symptoms in children. Too, it is possible that a latent but moderate case of TS was brought to the surface by the aunt's sudden death. We know there had been strain between the aunt and "Robby's" mother; the family seems to have been somewhat dysfunctional.

The question has been raised whether the aunt molested the boy; there was also a major fight about money the aunt was "juggling." We know that unbearable strain can cause tourettic symptoms in children too, a common situation known as Transitory Tic Disorder, and "Robby" had more than enough stress at home. In any case, after the involvement of the Catholic Church "Robby" certainly took a turn for the worse before improving.

Another example of the TS-possession link is the 1928 exorcism of an Earling, Iowa woman. This poor lady (whose identity has also been kept secret, and who is variously called "Anna" or "Emma" in the literature) began manifesting severe coprolalia and violent motor tics sometime after the death of her father. It had been discovered that her father attempted several times to initiate incestuous relations with her, which she violently refused. It is thought that he had extensively abused her as a child, and that she had blocked these horrible memories from her mind.

Just before her father died, he spat on the priest who was offering Last Rites and cursed "Anna" for never capitulating to his desires. He expressed with his last breath the hope "that the devil would take her." Eventually "Anna," like "Robby," began to echolate religious figures, such as Satan and Judas. She mimicked her father and especially her late nanny, an abusive psychopath who had murdered her own children. This lead everyone to believe that Anna was not only possessed by demons but also by the spirits of those she knew who had "gone to hell."

These are very powerful examples of the way tics can "enshrine" life experience. In the case of Robby, he seemed to restrict himself to creepy voices such as those heard in the movies, and also echoed the voice of his deceased aunt—probably mimicking arguments he'd overheard years prior. Then he began "echolating" religious figures after the Catholic priests became involved. The main exorcist, Father Bowder, was a tough WWII veteran, and approached the case with total aplomb.

In Anna's case, it is significant that she primarily echolated Judas Iscariot, then her father and her nanny in successive order of occurrence. In Robby's case, the fights between his aunt and parents must have come to the forefront of his tics. In Anna's case, the everlasting curse uttered by her despicable father, and the oddities of her psychopathic nanny, echolated and perseverated for years. It is clear that, had these unfortunate people's actual words been documented, we would have had more or less complete life-trauma histories for each of them.

It is widely agreed that this poor lady, aside from the experiencing the Post Traumatic Stress Syndrome one would expect, suffered from severe TS, as did her father. Even priests, doctors and the authors who researched her story have agreed one hundred percent with this diagnosis. But in Anna's time, no one could have ever thought of Tourette Disease. Being a Catholic, Anna was immediately taken to a convent for the Roman Rite of Exorcism.

Although in any exorcism the participating individuals' identities are kept permanently secret, the Roman Rituus of Exorcism is well known, and spectacular. Just the thing that is required in the case of a sexually abused, tormented, Tourettic woman! Two priests were summoned and participated in the grueling exorcism, along with the nuns in the convent where she had been taken. One of the participant priests was my brother-in-law's uncle, Father Charlie.

Initially it took years for the Church to decide that she was possessed, after all other treatments had failed. But this was standard practice for the Church, as it remains to this day. Considering the absolutely horrid jumble of symptoms that assaulted Anna, including all sorts of mechanical and animal noises, it is no surprise that the devil was blamed. Her violently explosive tantrums frightened the nuns, who were often overpowered by Anna in the throes of her worst motor tics. Years after the fact, nuns and others remembered "supernatural" feats of strength which, of course, never took place—though it is not difficult to believe the nuns who testified that poor Anna actually climbed the walls more than once.

And here again we have a happy ending. After the exorcism, which lasted from the end of September to sometime just before Christmas, "Anna" was successfully "exorcised." On the last day she jumped up from her bed, shouting in succession the name of each "spirit" that "possessed" her as it "left" her body, and loudly praised Jesus. (My brother-in-law's uncle, of course, never mentioned the incident; I learned of this through official documents in the possession of the Church and my brother-in-law's family.)

Significantly and not surprisingly, unlike Robby, Anna had been plagued with tourettic and post-traumatic symptoms since the age of thirteen, and had been exorcised several times before.

These links between echo-tics and possession have fascinated many people over the years (too many, I think). TS patients often speak and write of feeling possessed, and I myself went through a period convinced that Satan was after me (but I never, ever felt "possessed," though I can easily understand those who do). Dr. Tourette was fascinated by the "possession link," and wrote quite a bit about it. If I am not mistaken, it was Tourette who indicated that all documented cases of demonic possession were actually TS. He even wrote a play about Father Urbain Grandier, of Loudon, France, who certainly suffered from TS. (I believe the play is titled either "The Possessed," "The Devil at Loudon," or a combination of these two.)

Father Urbain Grandier, a 16th century Catholic priest, had been sent to a convent to investigate the bizarre goings-on. It seems that the nuns had gotten into some bad bread or mushrooms, and the result was something like mass hysteria. There was a lot of sexuality to their behavior; the nuns were masturbating and having sex with one another right out in the open, in broad daylight. Well, an entire convent full of nuns possessed by the devil had to be investigated! Father Grandier was sent; he was so overwhelmed that he suffered a severe exacerbation of his Tourette symptoms. This happens often: whenever a TS sufferer sees or experiences the wrong kind of stimulus, it instantly makes his own symptoms increase dramatically. There is no doubt that in the cases of Robby and Anna, this is exactly what happened.

The bishop discovered that Fr. Urbain was also going bonkers; he immediately accused the poor priest of being in cahoots with the nuns, and all of them being in league with the devil. Poor Father Urbain was immediately cast into a monastic prison, where he wrote heartbreaking, lucid and intelligent letters to his niece. These letters are absolutely sad and gut-wrenching, showing the priest as a compassionate, intelligent man who was convinced that he would be released one day. He never was, and was in fact burned at the stake along with the silly nuns. Fr. Urbain Grandier's story is one of the most famous of the Spanish Inquisition, and was eventually made into a film starring the late Oliver Reed.

Pretty scary, don't you think? Also not good for PR. Yet there is alot to be said for such reactions as these toward such severe symptomology, because it really addresses the seriousness of TS symptoms. Also, it is common for TS sufferers to exhibit full-blown Post Traumatic Stress Syndrome, and this does not mix well with any neurological disease. After exhaustive research in the field, and having performed exorcisms myself as a Buddhist priest, I am now certain that probably upwards of 99% of all exorcisms in the 20th century alone involved nothing more than severe Tourette's Disease. Interestingly, the better known cases show a classic history of tourettic symptoms, and most cases appear to have been triggered by some enormous stress.

This severe echophenomenal symptomology, which in its ugliest form is the essence of the classic demonic possession scenario, is obviously a horrible experience, unlike the seman-tics. It happens for no reason I can understand, other than stress and perhaps anger. It's very much like Dr. Morton Duran, the TS afflicted surgeon mentioned in a previous section, has said: "there is only the thinnest layer of cortex protecting us from the raging subcortical storm." The layer doesn't work too well for TS patients.

It goes beyond embarrassing for me, especially when speaking to strangers, but I'm happy to be able to suppress it most of the time. I tell my friends to make sure it's me on the phone when they call, as they might not always recognize me. My relatives, however, have almost all my "voices" down pat, so they know it's me even when I answer in another language.

Then there is a rather severe and distressing symptom present in Tourette Disease, one that would have assuredly convinced even an educated physician that the devil might be involved:

I Swear!: COPROLALIA

I use big letters because this symptom has been made into a big deal. This is the "swearing" tic, the first symptom that really brought TS into the modern layperson's mind. A common name once used for Tourette Syndrome was "Cursing Disease," and "Curse of Tourette's" was common also. Too bad those old-timers weren't inclined to a more African approach: the Zulus call Tourette Syndrome "The Great Pulsing." It is one of several sacred diseases showing the Gods' favor. Anyone with TS is chosen to become a king, a chief or a medicine man. We should not be too shocked to learn that coprolalia seems to occur statistically more often among the Zulus than any other population. Anyway, coprolalia can also involve racial slurs, inappropriate or disgusting remarks, or any conceivable obscenity.

It is uncertain exactly what percentage of TS patients have this vocal tic. America has settled on a figure of less than 30%, although this is in contest (I don't agree—I think it's extremely prevalent). In some cultures it doesn't really exist as such, either because the language contains no true obscenities (as in Japanese) or because social protocol is highly important (again, Japan, or the Muslim countries).

Dr. David Comings of City of Hope clinic has estimated a coprolalia statistic of around 40% in the United States. It is because he includes such manifestations as swearing at an early age and lifelong, habitual swearing if it is involuntary. This line of thinking jibes very well with what has been observed, in my opinion anyway. Especially in America, I think it is almost guaranteed that coprolalia and other copro-tics are going to go unnoticed (if not extremely severe) due to the growing use of obscenities by the general population. Certainly in the West's past, this symptom was the main cause for the calling of a Catholic priest to do his duty.

Well, in any case I have this awful symptom and there's nothing anyone can do. At least I'm usually not horrendously loud and explosive like some unfortunate sufferers are. Obscenities pepper every sentence I utter, unless I'm in a very precarious situation and really have to reign in my "exuberance." I suffer more than usual from this symptom when I'm suddenly irritated or startled, but it takes a fairly astronomic amount of sudden irritation.

As a small child I swore lustily, like a sailor (which I was, later in life) and no one could ever figure out how I learned such words. In any case I had my ears boxed more than once for this symptom; I've been routinely castigated and humiliated for it as an adult. The strangest thing is that it has become a sort of joke for foul-mouthed people to be thought to have, or claim to have, Tourette's. At least the disease is finally being acknowledged.

There are other tics in this category, called "coprophenomena." Such tics as constantly thinking or writing dirty words, or making obscene gestures, fall into this category. Dr. Bernard Simkin, whose name you will see later, wrote a paper called "Mozart's Scatological Disorder." It appears that Mozart loved obscenities, and he spoke and wrote them whenever he could get away with it. This tendency of Mozart's caused him no small trouble in society; the anecdotes about his childish scatological behavior, along with his letters, have lent support to Dr. Comings' research. It is precisely because of copro-tics and other inappropriate behaviors that an unusual strategy has been proposed to help deal with tourettic symptoms:

Tic Substitution

This brings us to the topic of tic substitution, which I mentioned some pages back. If a tic such as coprolalia gets to be too much, the TS patient is urged to try to "substitute" it with something different. For example, I make kissing noises which would be unacceptable anywhere in public, except perhaps when directed at a mule (or an attractive person), so I am able to substitute it with whistling or pursing my lips. This has made me wonder whether some folks can actually substitute a vocal tic for a motor tic, or vice-versa. I know I can't.

Even if tic substitution is a marginally possible coping skill (which I doubt), it doesn't mean everyone can do it with ease, or even at all. My personal opinion on substitution is that it is too much for anyone to ask of an already beleaguered Tourette sufferer. It amounts to asking the patient to control or manipulate the tics, which is the same as asking someone to stop any disease symptom by sheer will alone. This is because, as we know, the nature of TS as others wrongly perceive it makes them believe that the symptoms can be stopped at will.

Of course, Tourette sufferers become masters of symptom camouflage, and this actually can make the symptoms invisible at times. We can make a tic look like part of our true inner state, a comedy routine, bewilderment or anything. Have you ever become self conscious after doing something clumsy or silly, then pretended you meant to do it? We Tourette people end up doing alot of that sort of acting. Contrary to the learned, studied professional acting, we do it instinctively, of necessity.

If a tic is weak enough it will coalesce with the self and environment imperceptibly. Even if it's pretty spectacular, it can be made to look like something else, if the acting is good enough—and believe me it is! So if you're the acting type who is inclined to dream of polishing your hard-won Oscars, think about the TS patients: their burdens and how they have to be handled. *We* deserve plenty of Oscars (and your favorite performers don't act in order to psychologically survive. They do it for the money).

Related in an off-subject way to acting is something I've noticed in several films: the villains more often than not have some sort of tic. It reminds me of the days when the villains displayed homosexual undertones; but the tics are portrayed in an extremely obvious way. In one of Hitchcock's films the murderer, though in disguise, is easily identified by a persistent tic of his eyes. In one episode of *Star Trek: the Next Generation*, the android Data has an evil twin android, his "brother" Lore, whose identity is clearly indicated to the viewer by his facial and cervical tics. And who can forget the "Pink Panther" movies, in which the pitiable villain Chief Inspector Dreyfus (played with ferocious glee by Herbert Lom) is driven to Tourettic fury by the idiot Inspector Clouseau?

It's disgusting and unjust to think that the presence of tics indicates perversion, mental illness, criminal tendencies or worse. The truth is plain: people who suffer from TS are prisoners. Prisoners of a disease, of disobedient bodies, prisoners of school systems that refuse to help, prisoners of the prejudices and ridicule of others. We deserve to be out of prison! Not all of us are escape artists, and we shouldn't have to be.

If this unjust portrayal of a disease doesn't speak to the barbarity of our age, I don't know what does. It is tantamount to the old insistence that tourettic symptoms are proof of satanic activity. What is worse is the further link between the "possession viewpoint" and the fact that many serial killers claim that Satan directed them to commit crimes.

The Golem Has Tics, The Tics Are Golem

Anyone who saw the film *Backdraft*, in which there was much discussion about fire being a sort of conscious entity, will remember how chilling those scenes were. Tics are perhaps like that "conscious" fire, a manifestation of a sort of "lifeless lifeform" that seems to possess its own consciousness. In the same sense, tics could be thought of as "golem," a Hebrew word meaning "shapeless essence." The Kabbalist rabbis and scholars used the term to describe a Frankenstein-like clay monster, created by holy and well-educated rabbis. The golem, allegedly under the creator's absolute control and used to defend the Jewish people, usually becomes a raging monster.

Several golem stories (the best modern rendition of the classic is by Elie Wiesel), a modern film (*Snow In August*) and an old silent German film based on the German play "Der Golem," have been handed down to us, and the term "golem" still holds significant meaning for Jewish scholars. Almost all Tourette patients have stated a "golem" feeling about their tics. It must be added that it is precisely this very feature that makes tics look faked to the uninitiated. As if anyone would want to bother with such nonsense as faking tics! In other times, it was this otherness, this "mind of its own" aspect, which also made people suspect that tics were a sign of demonic possession.

You will recall that the majority of tics last a few months. The morphology of tics should be explained: tics can suddenly appear, can last anywhere from some weeks to several months (with a few being lifelong), and can mutate into a different tic or be incorporated into a complex "tic set" (such as the echopersonae). But then, it is just as likely that the tic will run its course, then vanish forever. After dissecting tic activity as we have been doing, this evolutionary trait in tics should come as no surprise. You could compare tics to a Lego set, though they are more like organic entities with a life of their own. Some of us would even say they have almost a consciousness, like a golem. At least you know you're Lego set isn't going to come alive and then mutate!

It would also be a good idea to briefly differentiate Tourette Disease from other illnesses that manifest tics: autism, Huntington's Chorea (which is terminal and has different symptoms), Wilson's Disease (too much copper in the liver), Sydenham's Chorea (a.k.a. "St. Vitus' Dance," a viral infection lasting about a year and considered to be a transitory, reversible form of Cerebral Palsy), Bell's Palsy, which comes from cold weather exposure and initially resembles a stroke, and other genetic diseases such as Rett Syndrome. Conditions brought on either by injuries or infections can also cause tics. But doctors are able to verify through tests and medical histories whether or not a tic is caused by any other illness or injury. Differential testing should be standard procedure in diagnosing Tourette Syndrome.

Rett Syndrome is worth a brief side bar here. It is a fascinating condition found almost exclusively in females; the genetic mutation of the suspected gene, which is on the X chromosome, is fatal to most males in utero or upon birth. Still I believe some males could have it, and I believe I have it. Rett is astounding because its symptomology involves autism, full ranging tics, OCD, and two exquisitely defining characteristics: tremors and constant hand-wringing. The definition of Rett Syndrome is basically a nutshell definition of my symptomology.

I seem to have been born almost externally hermaphrodite. I emphasize almost—not quite. There were the shots of testosterone I seemed to require from an early age, and one of my testicles (the right) never descended, and had to be removed. But I definitely am a male, even though it looked for the first few years of my life that my parents were considering raising me as a girl. I'm not sure why, and no one will discuss this matter today.

There is also the matter of my homosexuality, which is no source of embarrassment for me. I believe these genetic conditions may have provided me with the ability to survive the Rett's Syndrome genetic mutation, which is found on the X chromosome thus making it fatal to most boys. Today, doctors have discovered two characteristics that can allow boys to survive Rett Syndrome: either an XXY chromosomal structure, which allows for the extra X chromosome to carry the Rett mutation, or else what is called "mosaicism," in which the Rett genome is not everywhere in the body.

There is also the childhood condition mentioned in the chapter on demonic possession: "Transient Tic Disorder" which is said to affect most children. This condition manifests briefly with mild tics, and then disappears completely. There is also "Chronic Tic Disorder," which seems to be a sort of temporary Tourette.

Today, lots of doctors are looking at infantile strep infections as causes for these phantasmagoric tic- and autistic-variant diseases, which are collectively called Pediatric Autoimmune Neurological Disorders Associated with Strep (PANDAS). The boy who inspired The Exorcist, for example, could conceivably have had a form of chronic tic disorder due to PANDAS, since his symptoms were transient. Yet any of these disorders can baffle doctors as much as TS can. What upsets me is that although doctors often diagnose transient or chronic tics as anxiety, they misdiagnose full-blown TS as anxiety all the time!

Tics: Now You See Them, Now You Don't

However, to be fair to the doctors, there is a major detail about tics that needs further explaining. It is extremely common, especially with children, for tics to temporarily vanish at times. This can happen especially at the doctor's office. A TS diagnosis should involve a symptom history and the knowledge that tics can completely vanish, but doctors tend to ignore the fact that tics are rather sneaky. Whenever doctors don't see any tics, they will not diagnose TS when perhaps they should.

The matter isn't helped by the strange fact that Tourette sufferers CANNOT FAKE or replicate symptoms on command. It is virtually impossible for a TS sufferer to "perform" tics. All the doctor can do is elicit a detailed description of tic activity. One of the less intelligent books on TS suggests that the doctor monitor the children by video camera while they are alone. There is some merit in this, but the ideas of children and video cameras do not mix well in this criminal age.

I remember hearing many doctors remark that an absence of tics in the office is enough to rule out TS, and this is absolutely ridiculous. Richard Cytowic, the synesthesia expert, has complained about this very tendency among neurologists. As he points out, diagnosis itself begins with the patient's own descriptions and history. The doctor has to trust what the patient is describing, not just dismiss it as a lot of hooey. Cytowic uses the headache as an example: a patient complains about headaches, and the doctor will first try to find a cause.

Even if no cause is found, the pain is treated, because the doctor believes the patient really feels pain in the head. After all, why would a patient lie about headaches? Then a symptomological and medical history must be considered. Yet, Cytowic indicates, many doctors assume patients are lying or imagining things when it comes to difficult or bizarre neurological symptoms. He says this rotten habit that neurologists enjoy must cease, before any further neurological science research and development can flourish.

Tourette tics disappear for brief periods from day to day, and this also has been much described in the literature. Some of the literature states that tics occur throughout the day in bouts, but this is not true for all TS cases. When concentrating intently or participating in something the tics vanish, and this "lost tic time" does not need to be "made up" like a high school exam. As Dr. Sacks has noted, this also happens with Parkinson symptoms. I agree with experts that this is something like a re-routing of the neural misfiring which is believed to cause tics. I do not agree, nor do most TS sufferers, that tics disappear during sex and sleep. They are in a somewhat slowed mode during sex and sleep—but they're there for anyone to see.

It was thought just a decade ago that tics vanish during and just after sex. It was also thoroughly believed that tics disappear during sleep, an idea that Dr. Tourette himself introduced. This is simply not true. In fact it is quite the opposite. Tics increase with strong emotion, as I said; none can be stronger than the erotic passions. (By way of some minor consolation, I've had people tell me that some of my tics are sexy.) As far as sleep is concerned, most TSers can't fall asleep easily due to tics, though tics do decrease dramatically during sleep.

No one is sure why this happens, though I say it is obvious: the brain's asleep. It is said that the more relaxed we are, the more we tend to show symptoms. On the other hand, stress and tension will send symptoms through the roof. Speaking strictly for myself, my tics have 'minds of their own', and that's about all I know. One of the major themes that runs through Tracy

Hearle's Handbook for Parents of Children with Tourette Syndrome is the absolute avoidance of stress for TS patients. Easier written than done, Ms. Hearle!

In writing about Dr. Morton Duran, Dr. Sacks conveys the deep anxiety he felt when he observed Dr. Duran in surgery. At first he didn't know how Dr. Duran would get through the operation because his tics are very violent. Dr. Sacks noted with alarm that Dr. Duran had almost contaminated himself in the scrub room after scrubbing—not quite, but almost. Dr. Sacks, a very nervous sort, became increasingly nervous as he watched Dr. Duran tic his way through the entire surgical theater. Sacks continued to worry that Duran would contaminate himself because of his reaching/lunging tics. However, as soon as the operation began, Dr. Duran was completely tic-free and normal throughout the entire procedure. After the operation was over, Dr. Duran's tics resumed.

Duran describes this moment, when the tics resurface, as "almost 'remembering' I have TS, therefore 're-manifesting' the symptoms." Dr. Sacks noted the significance of one of Dr. Duran's "cardinal rules": he was never to be disturbed during surgery under any circumstances. In the past, Dr. Duran would be routinely disturbed, as all surgeons are, by all sorts of issues, questions or requests. Dr. Duran put his foot down and said the patient comes first. Disturbances were having severe effects on the doctor's tics, and he didn't want his tics to end up killing a patient. Dr. Duran's difficulties with broken concentration, like all TS patients, represent the other side of the tic-suspension coin.

Actually, the concepts of tic suspension, interruption and remission are quite like the idea of clear electrical signal reception: the less interference, the clearer the signal. I feel that tics could be some sort of grouping of crazy signals (NO, I did not say we are crazy), which could be compared to interference. When concentrating on a task or some other thing, the signal becomes clear and there is no ticcing. Many of the best minds in the Tourette field seem to agree with this illustration. This is not necessarily always the case. I can think of many things that I absolutely love that set off my tics, such as attractive people, favorite songs, good humor, fun events. It is true that strong emotion sets off tics every time. As I have mentioned, the mere thought of tics, TS, or watching another "ticqueur" can also lead to exacerbations.

You have seen that it is tough for us as TS patients, who sufferer from a hereditary neurochemical muscular movement disease, because the tics look so deliberate. They are strange, organic-like "entities," golems, shape-shifters that fly far above the ordinary concept we have of disease symptoms. I know too many people who just can't believe that tics are genuine symptoms of anything. In the strange turn of events we followed at the beginning of this book, we have seen how the earliest people to consider the nature of tourettic symptoms were well aware of their basic nature. Only later did the medical community fall into complete ignorance of outward tics and the nature of TS.

The Unbearable Interior: Internal and Emotional Tics

In view of the far-reaching influence of Tourette Syndrome and its tics, internal/emotional tics have to be addressed. Tics cannot always be seen or heard. I use the terms "internal" and "emotional" to run the gamut of tics that are not visible and therefore go unnoticed. There are other terms covering some of these types of tics, and we'll get to them momentarily.

Many more Tourette sufferers than you might think will go undiagnosed because they don't often show outward manifestations, and sometimes they never outwardly show symptoms. In fact it is often bandied about that men who suffer TS are the ones who demonstrate outward symptoms such as tics; women, the rumor holds, are more internally afflicted and do not show tics as much. It isn't clear how this rumor began, but I suspect that at most there is just barely a smattering of truth to it.

For starters, there is the simple internal tic group: the diaphragmatic contractions, the abdominal muscle "wave," the jiggling tongue, stiffening jaw muscles, excessive drinking of liquids (believe it or not!), biting the fingernails, wheezing, swallowing or gulping air, constricting the throat or anus. Tics such as drinking water or biting the nails have been only recently delineated; they could be considered gross motor tics.

I include them here because they are "internal" in the sense that everyone does such things occasionally, and they go unnoticed. Often, tics manifest in the various muscles in the hips and groin, the same muscles used in the sex act and to ejaculate. Sometimes these tics are painful. No part of the body whatsoever can escape the influence of Tourette Syndrome. Perhaps this will be the new definition of "tic" within the context of TS: "the involuntary influence on any part of the body and psyche that is caused by Tourette Syndrome."

Then there are the emotional tics: the bursts of anger, fear, depression, aggressiveness, elation, or amusement. Possibly these constitute a simpler set of Dr. Sacks' "tic of the whole personality." It isn't a matter of confusing them with our true emotions; it's that these tics are so overpowering. They are beyond normal emotional resistance, as involuntary and insidious as other tics. It almost seems like a sort of emotional immunovirus, in which the person suffers an attack from some weird, intrusive organism—in this case, a weird and intrusive emotion that is totally ego-dystonic. Again we have the intrusive organism theme—like the "possession" concept. I suspect that this type of tic is terribly common in autism.

"Mental" tics fall into the general category of "internal" tics. They plague me daily. As you will read in an upcoming section, it seems they may be related to obsessions—or that obsessions may be mild forms of this tic. I am inclined to believe the latter. They are very difficult to describe. I can only describe them as "jutting mind rocks" that one bumps into, falls on, scrapes across, sometimes splattering against them. You don't want them, you can't avoid them, they're not always there, and you can become quite afraid of them.

They are intrusive, perseverating thoughts which in extreme form remind some doctors of paranoid schizophrenic ideation. Mental tics are also ego-dystonic, meaning that they are the sort of thing the person who suffers them would never think, for any reason—they go against the person's very ego. In defense of some physicians, I have to say that it is the nature of these inner tics that is probably responsible for the occasional misdiagnosis of temporal lobe (psychomotor) epilepsy.

Another term I've recently seen in connection with mental tics is "Precipitating Preoccupation," which I believe describes a definite type of mental tic. It is a sort of avoidance "phobia," i.e., avoiding the outdoors for fear of rain when it looks cloudy, or avoiding interstates for fear of wrecking the car (this is my particular fear). Incidentally, this symptom also is found quite uniformly in all types of autism, and I will come to this topic again in the section on autism.

Dr. Sacks has written that many Tourette patients have a hard time driving because they feel other cars are too close, going too fast, or veering at them. I know I've experienced exactly this disorientation, and I think it is this that scares me, and not the driving itself. One of my former neurologists suggested that this difficulty driving was nothing more than banal obsessive compulsive behavior, but I disagree strongly. This kind of "precipitating preoccupational tic" does not fit into the fabric of plain OCD, but though examples of it are seen in OCD, I still believe that it is tourettic tic behavior not "obsessive compulsive" in nature.

Maybe the following example of my precipitating preoccupation about driving would best illustrate these almost unclassifiable tics: when I'm about to drive on a road I don't like, I experience a mental/internal tic. It is a tic of fear, but fear almost inconceivable to normal people. I can see the car going out of control, hear the wreck, feel myself pinned to the steering wheel, bleeding. It's ugly, but I don't always experience this scenario play in my mind—but I do always get the emotions connected with it.

So I don't really fear the road, my car, the possibility of danger or the act of driving. I fear the tic, and it's one tic that can't be substituted or treated in any way I know. It interferes with my driving ability much more than the motor tics do. The "precipitating preoccupation tic" is definitely not a classic anxiety symptom or phobia, either, though it could easily be confused for one (are you getting all this, my little physicians?). It is a great deal like the overcautiousness of plain OCD, but should not be confused with specific OCD symptomology as many doctors have done.

I've gone through periods with only internal, emotional or mental tics, and I know many TS patients experience this remission of external tics accompanied by torturous internal tic bouts. Added to this living nightmare is the fact that alot of doctors tend to ignore these symptoms, which they see as boring and prosaic, in favor of the more sensational and interesting symptoms.

Doctors should really not kick someone out of the office with a diagnosis of anxiety just because no simple-simon tics are manifesting at that moment. We've already got enough on our hands dealing with the innate spookiness of tics. We don't need noncomp professionals trying to tell us it's all in our imagination. If there's anything that's more Twilight Zone than Tourette Disease, it's those weird doctors who won't pay attention, who disbelieve anything their patients say.

A Brief Glossary of Tic Terms

Finally, I'd like to end this section with a glossary of tic terminology. It might serve as a nice overview of what has been a rather complicated section. It will serve you well if you are researching other TS literature.

Blocking- Stopping suddenly while speaking, seemingly "stuck" on a particular word. Has nothing to do with memory trouble.

Coprolalia- A tic involving the utterance of obscenities or other inappropriate language.

Coprophenomena (a.k.a. scatological symptoms)- Any symptoms dealing with obscenities of any kind.

Copropraxia- A tic involving inappropriate or obscene touching, of self or others, or obscene gestures.

Diaphragmatic/Laryngeal Chorea- Dr. Trousseau's original terms for vocal tics.

Echolalia- A tic involving the echoing, mimicking or repeating of others' speech or words.

Echopersonae- A complex tic involving the 'assimilation' or mimicry of an entire personality.

Echophenomena- Any tic involving any kind of imitation or mimicry.

Echopraxia- A tic involving the physical mimicry of others.

Emotional tic- A loss of control or surge of emotion.

False chorea- Dr. Bouteille's original description of motor tics.

Ideomotor- A term commonly used early in the 19th century to describe any involuntary tic-like movement.

Internal tic- A tic that is not necessarily visible as it involves inner muscles such as the abdominal, mandibular or rectal muscles. May include precipitating preoccupations.

Jumping (French Jumpers)- A manifestation of Tourette symptoms that seems limited to severe startle responses and a type of jumping.

Latah- The Malaysian word for TS. Manifests primarily with echophenomenal tics.

Mental tic- A "tic of the mind," viz., very similar to perseverating thoughts and obsessions.

Motor Incoördination- Dr. de la Tourette's original term for motor tics.

Motor tic- Any tic involving movement.

Myriachit- Sibero-Russian word for TS. Manifests mainly as echolalic and echopraxic tics, with severe startle response as a feature.

Palilalia- A tic involving the repetition of one's own words or speech.

Palipraxia- A tic involving the repetition of one's own movements.

Tactipraxia- A tic involving any kind of touching, with any part of the body, not necessarily obscene or improper (differs from copropraxia).

Vocal (Phonic) tic- A tic produced by the otolaryngeal system, producing noise or sounds. Can include speech of all kinds, mimicry, sniffing, coughing, throat-clearing and so forth.

Family and Reactions

Be strong. Be lamps unto yourselves.
-Lord Buddha's last words.

I clearly recall a phrase I heard throughout my childhood, and sometimes I even say it to myself: "Goddamn it! STOP THAT!!" It was the only phrase I heard with regularity, other than "What's wrong with you?" To this day these phrases continue to reverberate in my head, and from the mouths of people who should know better. I was considered an odd child, troublesome and frightening to some but charming to others. At times I could amuse strangers with noises, cartoon voices and accents, or frighten them by impersonating them perfectly. It was thought that I might be mildly autistic because of these characteristics combined with my status as a prodigy and occasional bouts of painful shyness or silence.

My family members wore themselves out trying to discipline me for all my symptoms (sounds like a soap opera: *All My Symptoms*). They were confronting me every minute about my behavior, tics, gestures and hyperactivity. I could no longer pass for an eccentric gifted child. Bear in mind that there wasn't a name for most of the developmental disabilities during my childhood years, and a comprehensive understanding of TS was still a desperately hoped-for event yet to come. The word "autism" was used only for Kanner's profoundly retarded, hopelessly disabled cases.

In a sense my total lack of comprehension was helpful: I became aware of how I looked to others, and my self control was helped by this knowledge. But I remember a junior high band trip, which I think was to a state competition (I play several instruments). As we sat parked, kids from another school in the bus next to us were laughing at me, saying I talked like Bugs Bunny. The worst part is that even today I sometimes talk like Bugs Bunny, as my voice tics its way into the higher pitches. Knowing how I appeared to others made me hate myself, a characteristic that has not entirely disappeared.

When I used to flap my hands or gesture, I got into heaps of trouble. One of my relatives made a remark using the word "faggot." At that age I had no idea what the word meant; today I HATE this word. My childhood, like those of most people with TS, was one of endless reprimands and punishments. I wound up feeling that no one liked me at all. I became very sensitive to others, picking up on their attitudes toward me and behaving accordingly.

This in turn caused an awful withdrawal, and for years I seemed to be nothing but a ghost, or one of those little lab monkeys who is raised in a cold, empty cage. Quite strange, really, when one considers that autism is supposed to create a perfect, inhuman isolation. Autism in truth does no such thing; for me, it certainly didn't—it only caused me to take others too seriously and worry excessively about what others thought of me, how they viewed me.

These kinds of things should never happen, should never be done to any child, yet I see it everyday when I'm around children who are with their parents. I want to slap those parents sometimes, then hug the kids and tell them it's OK. It's not right for parents to mercilessly bully their children; even more disgusting is the fact that it happens to adults at the hands of other adults. Everyone tells me that these negative reactions are natural: people fear what they don't understand. But the problem I have is with people who do understand, but they do it anyway!

When I was first diagnosed, most of my family refused to hear of it. After all, they thought, hadn't I always been a "problem" child, an "attention seeker," and a genius on top of it all? It's odd how they interpreted the reactions of others as being attention-seeking on my part. They basically thought I had somehow influenced the doctors to diagnose me for the sport of it. Paradoxically, they also thought I might be lying for the shock value, or that the doctor must have been "one of those worthless psychiatrists" (I do agree that psychiatrists are worthless).

Though I enjoy pranks that are harmless, pulling some sort of stunt for shock value is something I've never done—it's against my moral outlook and always has been. Tourette's Disease can make the sufferer seem like a kind of charlatan or liar, I guess. My family nurtures the attitude that such a thing as TS could not be an actual disease. They certainly nurture the idea that I am a charlatan and a liar.

When I was compelled to confront members of my family one at a time with my confirmed, formal diagnosis, they simply replied that I and my doctors were full of bull feathers. At most they felt that my trouble was a pathologically overactive imagination. Today, if some of my family members were to be asked what Tourette Syndrome is, they would respond that they don't know. They would behave as though they were being asked about the realm of UFOs, faeries and trolls. The sad fact is that such people will not acknowledge the truth: that TS is anything but a faerie tale. In reality it is a disease and it is a nightmare.

During my research I discovered that culture plays a role in how TS is perceived and manifested. The ancient Greeks viewed it purely as a physical malady. We've already gone over the Medieval Europeans' view—they saw it as demonic possession. American Indians and many other native cultures see it as the gods' favor; all Zulu kings, chiefs and shamans are chosen from among the sufferers of "divine" Tourette Syndrome. In many cultures it was thought to be some sort of weakness of character coupled with unspent nervous energy (a theory to which my late mother thoroughly subscribed).

To Mahayana Buddhists, its uninhibited, unconventional nature can represent complete mastery of the universe: if you can master the suffering of such a physical state, you can master anything. Tourettic enlightenment! It is strange, isn't it, that Tourette Syndrome is always believed to be anything other than what it really is? Or as eloquently put by one patient, "people are always suffering from my symptoms."

Finally I arrived at an explanation for my family's attitude. It's largely socio-cultural. They all manifest symptoms of TS to some degree: there are full-blown but mild cases, and some have autistic features, proving it to be genetic. In fact I can think of only one symptom-free person from every generation in the six generations of my family of which I have direct knowledge. The genetic aspect of TS has been exhaustively investigated by Dr. David Comings at the City of Hope Clinic in Duarte, California. His results are conclusive: it's genetic.

Anyway, I now believe that my family went into a panic when they heard certain characteristics of themselves being described. My family is one that has thrived and survived on denial. A family member who has a full-blown but undiagnosed case said to me, "Hell, that [the symptoms] is stuff that everyone does!" My father, who is severely affected by various tics and an autistic personality, dismissed TS as "one of those fantasy diseases that doctors dream up. It's nothing but the bad habits of spoiled brats!" These attitudes constitute a very sad sort of denial, and it's understandably common even among diagnosed TS patients.

These bad views lead Tourette sufferers to feel very guilty, as though everything were their fault. Negative views and ignorance can make entire families feel guilty, hostile and callous; this is strengthened by the fact that several family members will recognize TS or related symptoms in themselves when they learn of someone's formal diagnosis. There is a great deal of denial, of fear, running away, and evil behavior toward the afflicted person—the whole spectrum is there. It's no wonder people of old used to blame the devil—and the patient.

A lady publisher who agreed to read an earlier draft of this book sent it along to a good friend of hers, in order to get an insider's reaction; this friend has a son with TS. The publisher shot back the manuscript along with a letter. She didn't want anything further to do with publishing this book, because her friend had been frightened by what she had read.

She wrote to me that her friend had not wanted to even finish reading the book, because she thought I had so many things wrong with me that she didn't want to know any more—as if this book had some sort of power over her son! A more asinine and denying attitude I have never experienced, and that along with the humiliation of having my book rejected because it had too much information.

A woman of my acquaintance, who also has a son afflicted with TS and who encouraged me in the writing of this book, has a theory about why denial and ignorance are so prevalent among TS families. She said, "When your child is born you're handed this perfect baby...you want this baby to be perfect, then someone tells you something's wrong! Why, you can't believe it. You won't believe it!"

At the time, it seemed to me an overly dramatic thing to say. But now I can appreciate the profound truth in my friend's remarks. TS patients feel this way about themselves, too. Certainly my acquaintance was describing how she felt when she learned of her son's diagnosis; that was a painful day for them both. But as I told her, it is harder on the children to live in an atmosphere of choking denial. It is unjust.

Mere ignorance can be excused, I suppose, but the TS sufferer self-stigmatizes enough without this awful conspiracy of denial to cause the wounds to fester. It isn't enough to face the public, the doctors, the teachers, the acquaintances who will ostracize, poke fun, discriminate and scream. And there are other terrors to be faced when we're out among the ignorant...

Trouble In Paradise: The Police

I just can't believe it. I can't see how I would ever be able to believe it.

-A mother remarking on the arrest of her 8 year-old son, due to a TS symptom flare-up at school

There are quite a few stories about TS patients having trouble with the police. Tics and other character traits have often lead to trouble with our cities' finest. There are many heartrending stories of law abiding teens and others being dragged to jail for disrespecting or assaulting officers, all due to TS symptoms. Many severe Tourette patients can tell stories of spending at least one night in the drunk tank, stone cold sober, because of their tics. I personally know of a peaceful, thin young man who was dragged away in cuffs because he had spitting and kicking tics.

Under what was for him the extreme stress of the officer's presence, the boy of course kicked at the officer and spat at him. This lead to assault charges. The saddest part was that this young man's lifelong dream had been to enter law enforcement. Another little boy I know, whose mother is quoted above, had the police summoned by his teachers because they didn't know what else to do, in the face of a severe symptom flare-up. His poor mother practically flew over to the school, only to see her son in handcuffs, surrounded by police.

There have been special cards available for some years now, obtainable from the Tourette Syndrome Association, which identify the bearer as a TS patient. The card carries a brief explanation of Tourette symptoms and in large, bold letters states the involuntary nature of them. A TS sufferer can also custom-make TS cards; there are machines which can cheaply produce business cards. Also, a printer specializing in business cards might be willing to offer a special rate.

This advice goes hand in hand with getting a medical ID bracelet, tag or necklace. A wallet card with full statistics wouldn't hurt either; these are available upon request. TS patients should ask their doctor. Your doctor or neurologist should not object to helping out when something happens, especially with the police. In light of this, be certain to at least carry the business cards of your physicians.

Some time ago my credit union offered to make a credit card-sized medical data card; it has a tiny microfilm of a form that the patient fills out, and this can be read on the spot with a 4x magnifier. It can also be run under a microfiche machine. This card is to be carried at all times, and the company that made it for me also sent me a page of stickers. They say, "I CARRY A MEDICAL EMERGENCY DATA CARD IN _______," leaving a space for the patient to write in where the card is kept. I keep mine in my wallet. I placed these stickers around my car and on both my briefcases. Hopefully, this will at least give the TS patient and family a few good ideas.

I have often dreamed of suggesting to our legislators that people with Tourette and other diseases, which could be misunderstood and get into trouble, be issued special state medical photo ID's, complete with all the information anyone could need. But I suppose that idea smacks too much of police state tactics. After all, a card that clearly labels you as a disabled person… some might think it a step toward a Hitleresque philosophy.

I can assure you, I do not mean it in that sense at all. I have noted, by public poll more than anything, that most citizens strenuously object to the idea of a state or federal ID card of any type. Still, I think of how much trouble it would save if all citizens had such cards made available to them. Such cards could be initially ordered by the treating physician; the Department of Motor Vehicles could then provide the cards. Here in Illinois, special disabled persons' ID cards are available, but I just don't think that is enough.

We have to remember the police officer's duty, the fact that officers don't know for sure if they're going to make it home after their shift, or wind up in the hospital or in a body bag. When they encounter anything out of the ordinary, they will tentatively assume the worst: that the person is drunk, high or psychotic. This may be due to a lack of sensitivity training, but the truth is that the average officer doesn't see TS patients that often.

He or she has to be extremely careful; carelessness could cost someone's life. Afford the officer at least a slight chance to err on the side of caution;

often they begin their shifts with trembling knees, because they don't know if they're going to make it to the end of the day alive and unhurt. These facts are enough to warrant the TS patient taking proper and thorough precautions.

I've opted to suggest doing whatever seems comfortable and adequate, with a few exceptions upon which I insist. For the time being, we can each do something toward the cause of full and proper identification for TS patients.

Here are some pointers, which I've developed and practice conscientiously:

1. WEAR A MEDICAL ID OF WHATEVER KIND YOU WISH, BUT WEAR ONE!

2. Carry a detailed wallet card; be sure it also includes a "who-to-call" number.

3. Have someone reliable that the police can call; also have the numbers of your physician(s) on that card.

4. In the event of a mix-up with police, security or whatever, try to be calm and not talk too much. Come up with a SHORT script you can use in such a situation, and let the medical ID, wallet card, doctor and "who-to-call" lists speak for you.

5. The Tourette Syndrome Association has little information cards available that you can carry and hand out—you might order a few.

6. Above all, be gracious and patient. Officers and others really don't know who you are. They need you to give them the chance to find out properly.

Don't feel discouraged by the thought of dealing with the police. It will happen one day, whether positive or negative in nature. You as a TS patient must be ready. Try to have your family and friends prepared as well. It isn't a bad idea to promote or push for sensitivity training for police departments. My good fortune lies in the facts that I once worked in law enforcement and I know quite a few of our city's finest.

Thus I am also well acquainted with the circuit court judges here, and they all know about my TS. In fact, one of our prominent district judges suffers from TS. Often I used to be recognized due to the newspaper and television interviews I gave some years back. Even so, I never chance it—I have all my information on my person at all times. Of course I also stay away from trouble.

Naturally I can't do much if some over-fed, under-read loser is hell-bent on tossing me out of the mall, library or theater. This has happened to me quite often.

By now you will have me marked as a film buff. In that vein, I simply have to recount this story: when I was young I read Herman Melville's novel *Moby Dick*, and saw the film with Gregory Peck as Captain Ahab. More recently I enjoyed the excellent tv version, starring Patrick Stewart. Do I need to tell you that I immediately identified with the captain? I never knew why. All those years I struggled with my "dark side," I could identify with Ahab.

It even became a matter of echopersonae: I developed a limp where the "whale took" my leg. Oh, that white whale! It scarred my face! It took my leg! Damn it to hell, where I intend to send it as soon as I can find it! Well, I caught up with Moby Dick. That is why you are now reading this book. I hope you will read *Moby Dick*, or at least watch one of the two film versions. Meanwhile, think of this section of my book as the Piquod's log—and no one had to die!

My life has been luckier than some, I will admit. There is always someone around with whom I can share love, always the circle of friends who don't see the Tourette's Disease or the autism, but the True Me behind it. Some friends try to make life more fun by affectionately impersonating my symptoms in an effort to be closer to me. (This naturally leads to my echoing what they're doing.)

Even a few of my more hard-nosed relatives make it a point to mention whenever they've seen someone exhibiting Tourette symptoms, as though to comfort me with the information—which works. It means the family has seen some reason. I've always had people by my side, those who tell me, "I love you for who you are." If I could bottle that feeling and market it, I'd be Tourette's answer to Jonas Salk.

SECTION II:

ASPERGER'S AUTISM, AUTISM IN GENERAL, AND CHARACTERISTICS

The Shadow of Autism: Obsessive Compulsive Disorder

Though it is hardly necessary to add a book-length section on Obsessive Compulsive Disorder (OCD), I'd like to address it briefly for those readers who may be unaware of its full nature. Remember too that OCB indicates obsessive compulsive behaviors, and not the condition itself. This is a disorder which I believe is on the Tourette/autism continuum. The medical profession believes that it is an anxiety disorder; it may be noted that I have a very bad attitude toward anxiety disorders because I don't believe they exist. After all, every known disease causes a separate anxiety disorder in the sufferer, doesn't it?

Anxiety does not deserve a disease or disorder classification of its own, because too many doctors use it as an out whenever they are perplexed about someone's symptoms. A grossly disproportionate number of diagnosed sufferers of "anxiety disorders" wind up discovering that some other condition was the cause of the anxiety. The result is that the medical community has invented its own Judas goat so that they don't have to strain too much to make a diagnosis.

Also, I recently had an e-mail from a lady whose son suffers from a condition. The doctor prescribed a totally inappropriate medication for the boy, and the side effects were devastating. When the lady took her son back to the doctor, he misdiagnosed the boy with an additional disease—and all along it was nothing more than side effects. It was wise for her to get a second opinion, which was what she did.

Well, now that I've cleaned my poison pen, let's have a look at OCD. The prime components of this disorder are obsessions, which are perseverating mental tics as far as I'm concerned, and compulsions, which are involuntary activities which I believe are complex motor tics. Added to these main symptoms are heightened anxiety, hypervigilance, irritability and mood problems. We will address each of the symptoms in turn, and I hope to prove that they are mild "shadows" of either tourettic or autistic symptoms.

I. What It Feels Like To Obsess

Perhaps a good kick-off for this section would be to expand on my Captain Ahab obsession. As a child I had seen *Moby Dick* time and again; it was my favorite movie until "Star Wars" came along. Whenever I watched Gregory Peck stride across the deck of the Piquod, with all the pain and limitation of his whalebone leg, with the white scar on his face, he always reminded me of myself. A few years ago, Patrick Stewart starred as Ahab in an excellent, accurate television version.

Now as I think back to those feelings I had, Ahab reminds me of all who are faced with physical and mental challenges: he will stride on the deck of that ship, he will fight, he will overcome anything. "I would strike the sun if it insulted me," he snarls. It is Ahab's strength that always dazzles me, and I wouldn't be surprised if Herman Melville meant it to be that way.

Ahab was a man obsessed. His obsession with the white whale was his driving force, his anima and his animus. He is no longer whole, no longer the strong family man of faith he must once have been. I always thought he must once have been a Quaker; now he is the ultimate Apostate, bent on exacting "justice" at any cost. Whenever I think of Melville struggling to create this character, I am always reminded of Nathaniel Hawthorne, upon whom Melville had a life-long crush.

Hawthorne was highly embarrassed by his grandfather. Hawthorne's grandfather had been a judge, and was responsible for the American pogrom against the Quakers. Hawthorne must have struggled all his life against the shadow of his idiot grandfather, and Melville surely picked up on it to help create Ahab. It is important to bear in mind that Ahab is aware of his obsession, that horrid demon that threatens his life, his crew and his ship. At one point he is almost delivered of the obsession, but it takes over again at the eleventh hour. I sometimes wonder if Melville was portraying a side of Hawthorne that few people would ever know.

Ahab is a lovely icon of Yin-Yang imbalance: he has that white streak in his black hair, that white scar, that white leg, that white whale. Then he has his black clothes, black hat, black eyes, hate-blackened soul. The idea that he might have been a Quaker at one time utterly fascinates me; at the beginning, a crazy old sailor named Elijah warns Ishmael: "Did ye hear about how old Ahab spat in the Communion cup in Valparaiso [Chile]? They say lightning struck him, cleaved him in two for it."

Quakerism is a faith that has a powerful Buddhist-like nature; but Ahab as we know him is a violent, lighting-struck, quasi-mystical, driven monster of a man, a man rent asunder, drawn and quartered while fully conscious. Ultimately the imbalance kills everyone except the schoolteacher and storyteller, Ishmael. It is quite a novel, and though I might be accused of being biased, I think everyone should read it. Especially people with TS and those who treat them.

As I mentioned, I think of Melville's love for Nathaniel Hawthorne. I make the connection because there are several key Quaker characters in *Moby Dick*, and I believe Hawthorne may have been a "closet Quaker." Melville must have known that Hawthorne's grandfather had been one of those evil characters who led the persecution of the Quakers in 18th century New England. He must have sensed the guilt Hawthorne felt because of this, a skeleton in the closet that pained and divided Hawthorne within himself.

In that state, Hawthorne reminds me of a person struggling with symptoms of illness. Hawthorne's excellent short story, "Young Goodman Brown," has a theme of loss of religious faith. The theme is based on Goodman Brown's awful, traumatic experience with the "Old Man"—the devil. Perhaps Melville knew this story well. It has an undertone of impending insanity, annihilation, disintegration of the self. This too is a fine work of literature, though very short, which I think should be taught in the schools.

I've often pondered Hawthorne's "Young Goodman Brown," and how I could relate to its emotions. As a teen, my problems began to mutate from those of a simply confused, weird and twitchy kid; it seemed to me that I was insane or heading that way in a hurry. In spite of this, my new adolescent self-consciousness served as a powerful restraint for my tics. Studies have shown that cultural influence can also help in controlling (or worsening) symptoms; the culture in which I was raised is emotionally oppressive.

You've probably guessed that all my oppressive restraint backfired in a way: it made my problems almost impossible to diagnose. In other ways it made me suffer from the disease more than I should have. Hawthorne's character, John Brown, suffers the same tortures in the story, and even when Brown meets the devil it is nothing like the horror of what has been happening to him emotionally. There are times when I think I am exactly like Young Goodman Brown. In the end, Goodman Brown becomes a hoary, paranoid old goat who refuses to acknowledge the terrible symptoms he suffers. He sees evil and guilt in all the people around him, and finally dies completely out of his mind.

I was able during my teens to substitute my socially unacceptable tics, but everyone thought I was a nervous wreck, probably as a result of this self-repression. By then I was suffering from what seemed to be panic attacks. (Of course, these were mental tics with the attendant obsessive reaction.) In any case I'd come to be convinced that I was a "nervous nellie" and I acted the part. That horrible, yawning cavern of odd feelings was swallowing me whole: I had violent outbursts of anger, sadness and depression (emotional tics, or a reaction?).

Everyone figured that this was not like me, and the rumor circulated in school that I was completely out of my mind or on drugs. The fear of losing my mind was constant—no doubt the secondary reason for my so-called panic attacks—and at times I had the eerie sensation of not being real. The stress of my self-restraint and denial was literally threatening to kill me: I became suicidal. The fate of Captain Ahab and Goodman Brown was coming closer.

What I was to be told a few years after this period offered some hope: I received a diagnosis of Obsessive Compulsive Disorder. It accompanies TS in approximately fifty-five percent of diagnosed TS cases and consists of two classes of symptomology: obsessions (which we have examined and consist of perseverating thoughts, feelings or ideas that are involuntary and frequent), and compulsions (involuntary ritualized acts of all kinds).

Compulsions help (they help me, anyway) to relieve stress and improve memory. They've served me well in my battle against my other developmental disabilities. Some doctors have lumped in a sort of subclass of compulsion, which they call "impulsiveness" (I call it "impulsion"). But obsessions! What a torture! Only when obsessions are redirected and handled well can there be any hope for the OCD sufferer.

Obsessions come in two forms for me: agreeable and disagreeable. It is that simple. When I became obsessed with Albert Einstein in high school, I studied his writings, his life and his public persona. I became an expert in his life and his field of physics; that is obsession. I also began dressing and wearing my hair like him, in the true tradition of echopersonae. Then of course there is good old Captain Ahab, and he filled me with the burning will to go on. These two fellows eventually defeated the Goodman Brown in me. All of this provided me with an odd, vengeful obsession about myself.

This may have been the origin of my suicidal feelings: if I can't catch this white whale, I'll die trying! It was an internal civil war. Then, too, some of these traits are probably autistic in nature. Temple Grandin has written eloquently about being profoundly impacted by the android Data from the series *Star Trek: The Next Generation.* She has written that Data's struggle to become more human, and his comical misinterpretation of human feelings, reminds her of herself. I believe Grandin is also attracted by the absolute obsession Data has with becoming human, because it reminds her of her own identical obsession.

I also suffer from what I call "mental videos": it's as if a video is popped into my head and I can't stop it. It can consist of anything horrendous, from accidents to torture or rape, and often involves loved ones. This is so painful and ego-dystonic that I am cringing as I write. It may be that my "mental videos" are forms of precipitating preoccupation. This symptom I am almost never willing to discuss with anyone. It makes little difference to me whether or not it seems important to anyone else that I discuss these difficulties at length; they re like war memories.

I will say that there is almost NOTHING that could be shown or said to me that would come near causing the distress these "videos" cause. Like my father, I can sit through the goriest of movies and laugh my head off at the worst scenes. Dr. Morton Duran has mentioned similar "mental videos," which usually have to do with the well-being of his two beloved sons. As we will see a bit later, this is probably a type of thinking that torments high functioning autistics as well.

Obsessing is good in a field of study or scholarship. Many people mistakenly refer to this as compulsiveness, but it is not the same. Becoming obsessed with a subject is what makes the sufferer learn that subject to perfection. Aside from theoretical physics and many other things, it has helped me learn ten languages and several musical instruments to varying degrees. Becoming obsessed with detail provides the drive to perfectly accomplish things. Being obsessive at home—about how things are done, where they belong, keeping neat and clean—would do any military barracks or Zen temple proud.

Admittedly, obsessions and compulsions can blur into each other, and into tics too. There may be a healthy obsession with a salubrious subject; then there may be a compulsion related to that subject which is not so salubrious. Many autistic patients are obsessed by the weather and this helps us in many ways. This may become a compulsion to stay inside when it rains. On the other side of the coin, there could be a compulsion to check things a certain number of times—and checking a gas stove three times before leaving home, for instance, can be a very good compulsion.

Here there must be added a point: many psychiatrists (whose very ideas I do not trust) lately embarked on a new delineation of OCD which I mentioned previously. They claim that "true" Obsessive Compulsive Disorder only involves fairly simple stuff, such as fear of contamination, constant hand washing, or the need to count. Anything more complex, they claim, is Tourette symptomology.

I think this addresses the difficulty in separating the tourettic from the obsessive compulsive, and shows how confused the "experts" can become... unless we patients tell them what's happening. I suspect that this new symptom-distinction process is also going to happen soon with autism. In fact it has happened already to some degree, with experts struggling to define what "autistic" really means, and how many degrees of severity there are.

II. What It Feels Like To Have Compulsions

We probably all know someone who constantly has to wash their hands like Macbeth, count things and then tell everyone what the numbers are, avoid stepping on cracks in the floor, stare at the stove for ten minutes to be sure it's off, or other similar "weirdness." Probably you have known someone who needed to check things three times in a row, or do something over and over til it was just right.

Perhaps it's someone who had to have things just so around the house, with no other acceptable alternative, fearing that disaster would strike if everything wasn't in its proper place. Perhaps it's someone who never deviates from a routine, or someone who simply can't stop doing what everyone thinks should never be done in the first place. You might know a fanatic neat freak.

Here we are entering the other half of Obsessive Compulsive Disorder: compulsions. These are so similar to plain motor tics (less often like vocal tics) that they are primarily responsible for making the experts think that OCD is the opposite end of the Tourette Syndrome spectrum. Perhaps compulsions are the most readily identified OCD symptoms. A person so afflicted generally feels compelled to do silly, repetitive or dangerous things.

A few people I know have to stop in traffic, pull over and look behind them to make sure they haven't run over some poor slob. (You might have seen Robin Williams do this in his film *Fatherhood*.) Of course they know no one has been squashed under their wheels, but in such a case it's the obsession with possibly running over someone that compels. There are so many compulsions that it would be a headache to list every single one; and you must not get the impression that a compulsion requires an obsession behind it. In fact, that's almost like the old idea that motor and vocal tics "required" one another.

The most common compulsions are neatness/environment-oriented: grooming, counting, checking, repeating oneself, stepping a certain way or on certain spots, hopping and twirling. As you can now see, the actual behaviors themselves are indistinguishable from tourettic motor tics. A compulsion feels like "home": it's a comforting routine that approximates superstition, a security blanket if you like, and a relief from obsessive thinking. At the same time it can be miserable, incessant but for its acting out, tearing at the mind like a mad Doberman pinscher. Or as Sherlock Holmes once said, "…like an engine that will tear itself apart..." Even the deliberate planning and thoroughness of the neatness compulsions have an almost involuntary, eerie quality that makes me suspect they are a sort of "slow motor tic."

The one major characteristic that compulsions share with tics is the lack of pure premeditation. They seem to me to be just as involuntary as tics, even though more planning and subsequent after-thought might go into a compulsion than into a tic. Notwithstanding that fact, it is in this sense that compulsions are very much like the twitching eyelids that some people experience in the winter, or trembling hands before a speech.

I'm afraid this is as close as I can accurately get at differentiating compulsions from tics; it's an area where everything gets really blurred. It seems clear to me that compulsions are probably nothing more than a form of complex tic. In any case, it is a fairly simple instance of a typical neurological pathology: something neurological happens that makes no sense.

This reminds me of those shows with hypnotists. The hypnotist takes a sucker from the audience and hypnotizes the person, planting a subliminal command. On one such program, the hypnotist told the poor fellow, "When you wake up, you will hear me say the word 'Well.' When you hear that, you will act like a chicken." Then the hypnotist brings the guy out of the trance. The hypnotist then says, "Well, folks..." and the poor guy begins clucking and flapping his arms.

Then the hapless victim laughs and says he can't understand why the hell he did it. Of course it's up to you to decide whether you believe in hypnosis itself; yet somehow the results of this kind of hypnotism reminds me not only of compulsions but of tics. It's like having been neurologically "hypnotized" in a sense, and it's an interesting harkening back to Chevreul's "state."

If you really want to go on a wild but beautifully accurate ride with compulsions and the relation to TS, rent Jack Nicholson's movie *As Good As It Gets* (1998). His character, Melvin Udall, suffers from Obsessive Compulsive Disorder, but if you look carefully you will observe that he also has Tourette's Disease and a touch of autism. It is really a fantastic portrayal, right down to the TS personality, with testing of social boundaries, blurting offensive phrases, and mimicking others. Nicholson is as good as Robert DeNiro is in *Awakenings*, and his portrayal shows the fuzzy line between OCD and TS.

If you pay specific attention to Nicholson's regular dialogue, which is offensively blunt and totally lacking in internal editing, you will see a very subtle type of vocal tic in action. You will also notice the classic tourettic aggressiveness, and if you look very closely you will see other subtle, tourettic tic-like behaviors. It was truly the Oscar-winning performance of Nicholson's career.

The beauty of the movie is that Nicholson's character, hated by all because of the obnoxious nature of his symptoms, "finds" himself with the help of two friends, Simon, a gay artist (Greg Kinnear) and Carol, a waitress (Helen Hunt). In the movie we see how the two friends, especially Helen Hunt's waitress character (and the gay artist's small dog), move Nicholson's Udall to finally understand and improve himself. What is sad is that the character has clearly had no substantial help from the psychiatric community and therefore doesn't want any—sound familiar?

In an amazing moment, Nicholson even illustrates the autistic features seen in TS. He enters his doctor's office without even glancing at his doctor, looks about the place in alarm and says, "You've changed your office around!" The psychiatrist caustically responds, "Two years ago. I also re-grew my beard, but you don't care about that..." Whoever wrote this character really knew his stuff.

In coming to understand himself through the eyes of his new friends, Nicholson's character finds a therapeutic situation in which everything is slowly scrutinized and finally understood. Hunt's character has a son suffering from severe respiratory troubles which disable him. Nicholson's character, in an attempt to gain what he wants, provides full health care for the boy which could otherwise not have been afforded. Later he reveals that he did this because he truly cares about the boy and the waitress.

In another scene, the turgid homophobia of Udall melts when the gay friend tells him he loves him. Udall replies that if he himself were gay, he'd be the luckiest man in the world. We see as the film progresses that perhaps Nicholson is also trying to give the waitress's son something he himself never had: proper attention and care. This is precisely what is so lacking in Tourette's, OCD, and indeed many TS/OCD sufferers show this tendency. With his heartfelt revelation to the gay artist, Nicholson's character provides the other things he never had himself: acceptance and understanding.

The gay artist, in demolishing Udall's self-centered, needless self-pity with his suffering, offers us another tender illustration: what true suffering is. It is through this character that Udall finally sees his own suffering—though very real—for what it really is. Udall is not suffering from dirty hands, or rotten people, or intrusions on his selfish wants. He is suffering from a disease, lonely, by turns alienated and alienating, wasting away as a human being. It requires the awful torment of a gay man right before his eyes to make him realize his true nature, his own true suffering. And it is in his initial attempt to reach out to the young gay man, whom he despises in the beginning, that he first learns what it is to care for another—and to heal little by little in so doing.

The waitress character Helen Hunt plays reminds me somehow of Jane Gooddall, the scientist who studies chimpanzees. Dr. Gooddall is such a fascinating figure. She has gone out to scrutinize these lovely animals, to understand them, to live with them and be part of their lives. (In fact, she seems to be compelled to study them.) Why can't more people do this with diseases, with sufferers and patients? Not to say we are chimps!... but we could use our own Dr. Gooddall, or at least a blunt, caring friend like Helen Hunt's waitress. I suppose if we examine and understand the combined efforts of Drs. Sacks and Comings, we'll have the closest thing we'll ever get to this ideal.

My other point in mentioning Dr. Gooddall is that the natural grooming and territorial behavior of the chimps reminds me a great deal of obsessive compulsivity. When I see the documentaries, showing the chimps grooming themselves with microscopic detail, behaving strangely, or carefully eyeing their environs, I am reminded of nothing so much as myself, or rather, my OCD. There is also a staggering similarity between some autistic and OCD symptoms and the behavior of other mammals. This animal quality probably points to a specific part of the brain involved with OCD and TS, perhaps a territorialist-survivalist portion that has atrophied in most people. Perhaps it's simply a counterbalance, with the brain trying to make up in some way for the disturbances caused by the disease.

I'd like to again emphasize that the line between tics and compulsions is fairly blurred most of the time. It is clearly easy to confuse them, as in the examples above. What is truly mystifying is that the tricyclic antidepressants used for OCD do not work at all on TS (or at least not as much as we might think they would). When I took imipramine (Tofranil) years before I was diagnosed with TS, it was to stop my night terrors and improve my sleep. But it took care of other problems as well: my jumpiness, fixations, irritability, aggressiveness and moodiness were all gone. But oddly enough, all the tics remained, completely unaffected. This taught me that tics are not anxiety-caused in the least.

What actually saved my life from the OCD trouble was Anafranil, another tricyclic antidepressant. I can't think of any other medicine as excellent as that (I've tried 'em all!) and the side effects were minimal. People with TS have strange side effects with all medicines; no one knows why. It has been said that whatever side effects a drug causes will be experienced differently by Touretters—in other words, whatever the side effects are, the tourettic person will experience the opposite.

I certainly suffer from weird side effects, even with over-the-counter items. Anafranil was terrific. When I went off it about eight months later, my OCD was eradicated. Only recently have I begun to show a few minor symptoms and some symptoms that I never had before; it's in the air at this point how they will be handled and why they returned at all. One thing I do know is that I can no longer tolerate tricyclic antidepressants or serotonin-reuptake inhibitors (SSRIs). I am now "allergic" to them all.

This part of the book should be concluded with a personal note, one that I think may offer new insight into OCD. Over the years I have noticed that my OCBs do not seem to really apply to my car. My car is neat and organized, but it is filthy! In fact I abhor the thought of cleaning or vacuuming it. I've had the trusty little Ford P.O.S. for ten years, and I've never cleaned the inside. Naturally I have done some interior window cleaning, and I wash the car regularly, a habit I picked up from my law enforcement days.

The inside of the car? It's basically ignored. I've wondered why my tendencies don't really extend to my car very much. I've concluded that my car is rough and ready transportation, subject to extremes that can never be controlled. Accepting that fact makes it easier to just hop in the car and concentrate on driving, when distractions cannot be afforded. It points up a vital characteristic that has never been addressed: obsessive compulsive behavior can be suppressed or suspended to a degree, the way TS and certain autistic characteristics can be.

III. Phobias

Usually one does not see much about phobias in Tourette, autism or OCD literature. They are worth mentioning because of the blurry line separating classic phobias from disease-induced phobias. There is a spectrum between the two types of phobias. Firstly, for the purposes of this chapter, we shall assume "phobia" indicates the disease-induced type found in TS, autism and OCD. For this chapter, we shall define "phobia" as any abnormally strong fear, revulsion, repulsion and/or avoidance of any particular thing.

It will behoove us to take baby steps in examining phobias, because the phobias themselves develop in baby steps, and very predictable ones at that. An autistic, for example, who does not like the sensation of getting wet may develop a phobia of thunderstorms, or even develop agoraphobia, which is the fear of leaving the home. People with Tourette symptomology frequently develop agoraphobia simply because they fear being seen, that is, being ridiculed or mocked.

Obsessive compulsives often develop some degree of agoraphobia because of other true phobias, such as the fear of contamination. But don't be fooled by the apparent complexity of disease-induced phobias; perfectly normal people have been known to develop such phobias as the fear of clowns or of the number 13! (Don't feel badly if you're one of those people.)

It has been my experience that a phobia begins when a deeply unpleasant symptom is experienced in tandem with a particular environment or activity. It is initially the fear of the recurrence of the unpleasant symptomology that causes the subsequent phobia of the environment or activity in general. I can speak to this immediately and at length, for this often happens to me. Of the few phobias I suffer, all are symptom inducement-related, meaning all had their origin in unpleasant symptoms.

Therefore I have phobias of high places (like Einstein, I almost fell off a mountain once), of spiders (I was bitten and reacted severely), of dogs (like Thelonious Monk I was mauled by a German Shepherd, but I was three), and of driving (I get motion sickness, which is quite an ordeal for me). To a certain extent I am xenophobic (fear of others), but that is purely due to their reactions to me.

A very severe phobia found in almost all afflicted people is conflict phobia. My own xenophobia is shared by most TSers, autistics and obsessive compulsives. There is no need to delve into the complex machinations of the fear of conflict. Suffice it to say that we have enough conflict without knowingly walking into some new, unexpected or sudden conflict. This is a truly problematic phobia, as most otherwise normal people who suffer from it can attest.

Its direct result is a failure to stand up for oneself, and from that follows a sort of crippling of the communication abilities. Then a mania (the opposite of a phobia) will develop, such as a mania for privacy, avoidance of people (not necessarily a fear of people) and so forth. In extreme cases, like with everything else, this phobia is the second leading cause of agoraphobia.

Conflict phobia—that is, the fear of conflict with others—is the most difficult to handle, especially in autistic people. My advice on the matter is to basically forget trying to monkey with this, if it concerns an autistic person. I believe this is the best course because any attempts to neutralize this phobia will in themselves produce conflict. It is a thorny problem, and the autistic person is the most susceptible to being pricked. My suggestion is that, in the case of the autistic, a family member or friend should help guard against and ward off any such conflicts. It is easy enough to have a member of the individual's support network to take on this small responsibility—normal people are not generally conflict-phobic. This is the only real case in which I advocate such a course of action.

This is not an attempt at mere sweeping-under-the-carpet. Autistics have more than enough trouble communicating, at least sometimes. Attempting to reverse conflict phobia will surely deepen the autistic behavior to a degree. Having said that, one other phobia comes to mind, which I myself suffered for the first half of my life: the telephone. This is a phobia of answering or speaking on the telephone, and is extremely common in autism and TS.

The only thing I can say about this phobia is that it should be handled in some constructive way. In other words, it should be dealt with head-on by the sufferer. The phone will not bite, and conflicts rarely occur over the phone. When they do, the magic bullet for this phobia is a simple one: hang up! Now, as to making phone calls, practice, write a script, do whatever it takes to learn to penetrate this fear. It is essential. I do all of these things in preparation for many phone calls that I have to make.

People are astonishingly rude and aggressive these days. They have no good reason or excuse. This can actually cause conflict phobia in those who do not have it. So I take the opportunity here to state that this rudeness and aggressive behavior must STOP. If you are one of the perpetrators, I have to ask, Why do you think it's necessary to be so mean to people? What will it cost you to do your job, be polite, be patient? You never know who you might have on the other end of the line.

There is a good, simple remedy for handling such people, and it occurs in two steps: be patiently stubborn about what it is you want, and if necessary, stop the conversation and inform the other person that he or she is being rude or whatever. Then resume pressing for what you need. It can all be done in a perfectly normal speaking voice, and it works wonders. Even autistics with relatively good communicating abilities will find this a pleasant, easy solution. Those who suffer speech impediments will at the very least find this tactic to be in essence effortless.

The fear of standing up for oneself extends to a total fear of communicating. Some have trouble asking for what they want, while others have trouble demanding action or making complaints. My above solution works well to neutralize all such fears. Just try it, try it one time, and be amazed at how effective it really is. You must force yourself to command the respect of nasty folks.

If you are unfortunate enough to encounter a persistently aggressive, uncoöperative bonehead, simply talk (or shout) over them until they are quiet; then tell them they are too rude to deal with, and that you will be having a word with their superior. End of conversation. No matter how mean they are, they know they're cut off, and they know they might be getting into some trouble. Never forget that everyone has a boss—and bosses don't like to hear that their employees are generating complaints.

Once in a while you'll encounter a person who simply tunes you out—even if you are in their face. This recently happened to me. Being ignored like that is a really easy dilemma to solve: just tell the offensive person it's fine if they ignore you. Tell the person it won't have anything but a worse effect on the trouble they'll be getting into. No matter how hard they try to ignore you, they still can hear you!

The detail I've supplied above makes a good template for handling most phobias. When we are facing our conflict phobia, we have to deal with other people in a rational, logical way. We have to ignore or fend off any irrationality. We must learn to do this when dealing with ourselves, too. Often I find myself angry at very high functioning Asperger sufferers, because they use their condition as an excuse to have it their own way all the time. Dr. Asperger was unfairly criticized for noting this tendency in his patients.

I have an acquaintance who suffers from AS; he is now successfully completing his freshman year in college and is a happy brother in a fraternity. Yet he will not speak to me on the telephone, and I have made it clear that I want to talk to him, not just exchange e-mails forever. He refuses, and plies his alleged lack of communication skills as an excuse. As of late he has simply ceased all communication with me, out of fear. Thus he will enable his phobia for the rest of his life—at the expense of others. Just as there is no excuse for others to be illogical, there is no excuse for us, either.

It's A MAD Disease:
A Brief Ode to and Lamentation for William ("Bill") M. Gaines

Though this chapter would at first seem to fit better in another section, I place it here because the man with whom it deals, Bill Gaines, identified himself simply as "a compulsive," but he was exemplary of Asperger's autism as well as OCD. He went from a boy who was considered a loser to the greatest humor publisher of all time. He went from being a hot-dog-and-Chef Boy-Ar-Dee-spaghetti-dinner kid to a gourmet. He went from guzzling Manischewitz wine to being one of the more important wine connoisseurs and collectors of the 20th century. He went from the inept son of the fellow who pioneered modern comics to a multi-millionaire in a little more than a decade—taking over the pioneering for himself. And he went from cranking out horror pulp comics to being the publisher of the greatest humor/cartoon magazine ever published.

The late Bill Gaines was the creator of "Mad Magazine." Bill's father, Max, was the inventor of the modern comic book and the creator of educational comics. Bill was most colorfully described as a "virtual snakepit of neuroses." Today it is clear that Bill suffered from autistic-type extreme obsessive compulsive behaviors; I have also found that Gaines was afflicted with Asperger's autism. He is a prime example of what an OCD sufferer is like, but also a good illustration of how autism can be deeply buried and hard to distinguish. Still, his magazine, his ideas and his life's work exerted a profound influence on me as they did on almost every American since the early 1950's.

Gaines followed a pattern of development similar to that of many mildly autistic people, especially Asperger sufferers. Early in life he was clumsy, quiet, and timid; later he became somewhat like his father: loud, brash, foul-mouthed and aggressive—but never overly so. Probably because he had finally found his niche after inheriting the comic business founded by his father, Gaines grew in confidence and eccentricity. It was not until this time in his life that Bill Gaines was "free" to live according to his strident, inflexible routines and obsessions. He charmingly referred to himself as "a compulsive" all his life, but unlike classic OCD, he exhibited no overt symptoms until his early adulthood.

Frank Jacobs, a "Mad" staff member and long-time friend of Bill's, wrote the book on Bill Gaines in 1972, called The Mad World of William M. Gaines. It is the primary source for this section, and is cited in the bibliography, in the autism section. From eyewitness accounts to his own experiences, Jacobs cleanly and hilariously outlines Gaines' "compulsions," as well as the great contributions Gaines has made to the publishing business. The book reads like a "how-to-diagnose" list. Jacobs' biography has become a sort of Gaines/ Mad Magazine bible.

Gaines enjoyed full and inviolate control over his environment, which he maintained at a most rarified level. He measured every item on his desk to be certain that every thing on it was equidistantly separated, from all the other things and from the edges of the desk. He had his cherished lists and a master list of all his lists; he had his narrow obsessions with food, wine, King Kong and zeppelins. He was a notorious slob in his personal appearance. Like Einstein, he gained a sort of fame on that basis alone: his hopeless beard and hair "styled only by the force of gravity" made him distinctive indeed.

Yet, like Einstein and so many others of us who are on the autism spectrum, Gaines had a system of buying, laundering and putting in order his clothes (and his life) that made him seem, in Jacobs' words, like a "poorly dressed Prussian." He purchased identical clothes in varying sizes to accommodate his fluctuating weight—no small feat considering that its average fluctuation was more than 100 LBS. Each size of every article of clothing had assigned to it a number for easy reference; a number 10 trouser, for instance, was good to wear when Gaines weighed around 250 LBS.

There was the matter of Gaines' apartment. With the celerity of a drill sergeant Gaines was truly the master of his domain. His father Max had instilled in him the old rule, "A place for everything and everything in its place." Gaines took it to its ultimate potential. Like autistic people, he knew if anything had been moved a fraction of a millimeter in any direction. He could tell when there was something in his environment he didn't like—his wife was incapable of sneaking eggs into meatloaf, which Gaines hated.

He could tell there were eggs afoot without ever giving his wife the chance to use them. He liked to see the cans of Campbell's soup arranged in alphabetical order, and bought supplies in threes, sixes, twelves, and multiples of twelve. As soon as one thing was used, Gaines would immediately go buy another, to keep his numbers balanced. He could tell when his wife tried to do something he didn't like—she said it was as if he had employed an "invisible private investigator" to watch her while he was at the office.

Gaines ran his magazine completely, with his own two hands. He insisted all his life that he should retain this total control; in his own words, he served as everything from stock-room boy to payroll master. He had two secretaries; one he kept because "she's the only one who knows how to open my safe." The other secretary he retained because the two made a good team, and Gaines hated the thought of breaking it up.

He protected his baby, which was also his family and his very identity; like all autistics who are able to function well, he needed and built a support network around himself. The magazine was his lifelong obsession, prompting him to become a business wizard. But much of what he did in apprenticing for that wizardry "no executive in his right mind would do," as he so eloquently put it.

Two highly essential items in Gaines' life were his calendar and his rubber-stamp rack, a large, old-fashioned circular carrousel that held dozens of individual stamps. Gaines could reach the brink of insanity if his daily calendar wasn't clean at the end of the day; sometimes he might fret for a week if he couldn't reach someone over the phone. Usually, the call was just to say hello. His closest associates, like fun-loving family members, would often threaten to hide his rubber stamps or overturn the rack. As is typical with autism, Gaines refused to buy a newer model rack; he refused even to buy a second back-up rack. Incidentally, one of Gaines' rubber stamps, with which he stamped the backs of checks received, holds the record as being the longest-worded rubber stamp in the world. It consists of an unbroken paragraph-length sentence of more than 185 words.

Gaines, like most autistics, was a compulsive list-maker. His lists were a large part of his life, and they were as cherished as any family heirloom might be. Gaines had lists of everything, except one thing: he had no master list of all his lists. After Jacobs proposed they sit down and calculate the number of lists Gaines consulted daily, Gaines kept the results as his Master

List. Jacobs calculated that Gaines maintained over 30 lists. He also had no compunction about building a special closet in his luxury apartment to accommodate his fine wines.

The temperature was kept at a year-round constant by an air conditioner that was never turned off. Yet Gaines would not order a separate phone line for his teenaged daughter, for fear of being "tied down to a $15 a month phone bill for the rest of my life." Similar behavior, albeit not quite so extravagant, is common in autism. Gaines was also well known as a skilled but gutsy, compulsive (or rather impulsive) driver. He seemed to court danger while behind the wheel, and often drove at speeds exceeding 100 m.p.h. This driving behavior, believe it or not, is also common to HF autistics.

Again like Einstein, the Jewish Gaines became an atheist at the age of 12. Like Einstein, he found it illogical that God could exist. To that end Gaines exhibited a lifelong abhorrence of authority—he was the type of boss who inspired respect through love and friendship rather than through force. His father had forced respect from those closest to him, and appeared to have had a form of ADHD, which is totally common in such cases.

Like many obsessive compulsive people, Bill had disturbing, intolerable sensations, such as the inability to eat steak ("When I cut a steak I am cutting flesh, and it disturbs me" he moaned woefully to Jacobs) and the fear of having his blood drawn. Gaines was labeled as phobic when, in fact, his "phobias" were clearly OCD/autism-related symptoms. For example, his greatest fear was the fear of invasion of his personal space and environment. This is not a phobia per se but a consequential symptom of autism and OCD.

Like Einstein and so many others, Gaines showed a bit of callousness and insensitivity toward others. In his case, Gaines loved practical jokes, and was an expert at playing incredibly cruel ones. Whenever his mother drove with him, she would demand to know why he had to drive so fast and recklessly. "Because I want to splatter my body all over the road," Gaines would respond in robot-like fashion. Never did he overstep the boundary to cause physical harm, though he certainly caused much psychological harm with his monkey-like pranks and sophisticated fear-inducers.

Only on one occasion did Gaines admit defeat. He had visited the house of friends for a dinner. Later he sent his host a note saying that he had hidden, somewhere in his host's apartment, one of the silver spoons from the silver set that his host's wife so dearly cherished. Of course, Gaines never took anything; he knew that all they had to do was count the silver and see for themselves.

The fellow proved to be Gaines' match. At first he sent pleading notes, saying his wife was not happy about her heirloom silver being used in such fashion, and would Gaines please tell them where the spoon was hidden? Gaines became perplexed and agitated; did someone else really lose or steal one of the spoons? Soon the fellow was sending Gaines hysterical notes about how badly the spoon was needed; he wrote Gains that his wife was about to leave him. With that, Gaines was finally forced to write the fellow a new note. "All right, you son of a bitch, you've got me. You win. I never hid a spoon," Gaines confessed. The fellow breezily laughed it off, having succeeded in making Gaines sweat for a change.

There was another incident that occurred much later: during the height of Gaines's fame, an enemy who knew his autistic traits used them to wound Gaines deeply. This person had taken to breaking into the MAD offices at night and stealing little things or petty cash. Once he knocked over Gaines' rubber stamp rack, scattering the dozens of rubber stamps all over the room. When Gaines had his fake diamond ring stolen, he loudly proclaimed it was really a cubic zirconia replica of his favorite, genuine diamond pinky ring. Gaines bragged that he had placed his ring into the safe and had the replica made the same day.

The thief, whom Gaines had named "The Phantom," was apparently enraged by the worthless ring he had stolen. When he broke in that night, he camped in the offices over the weekend; he obtained and burned files of Gaines' most vital papers—including priceless old comic book springboards, records, and his lists. As a parting gesture, he stole Mad's mail right out of the postman's bag! Jacobs said that Gaines was never the same after finding the leftovers of the little bonfire in one of the unused offices, and that he wept openly for the first time since his father died, over the burned lists and papers. No one ever discovered The Phantom's identity.

Like many autistic people, Gaines had made up his mind at one point that he knew exactly who The Phantom was. Gaines had phoned everyone one night when The Phantom struck, and only the one employee was not at home. Of course, Gaines was wrong, and was profuse with his apologies. But it is truly odd that someone who knew him so well, so intimately, could do such a terrible thing. Everyone who knew Gaines loved him (with a few business exceptions, naturally). Gaines was a boss who earned respect easily, was generous to a fault, and treated his employees like his own family.

The Phantom had to be an inside job—the worthless cubic zirconia ring was the only thing the vandal ever tried to steal that was of any solid value, aside from the petty cash. Then, The Phantom immediately knew that the ring was a fake when Gaines loudly bragged about it the following day. Whoever The Phantom was, this was no practical joke as Gaines might have thought at first. This person had struck Gaines a mortal blow.

The Phantom forced Gaines out of his beloved old offices. As Jacobs pointed out, Gaines was never the same, and his phobias, paranoia and uncompromising routines became even more hard and fast. Gaines had, in fact, descended a bit more deeply into his autism, and the entire staff suffered to a degree. The employee whom Gaines had initially (and wrongly) suspected immediately suffered a nervous breakdown. Gaines became very security conscious, and in very short order became security obsessed, really overdoing it.

It was to be expected that some of the staff would quit; Gaines would immediately have quitters investigated, in the futile hope of finally learning The Phantom's identity. Some of those disgruntled employees simply balked at Gaines' excessive paternalism, not appreciating the control he seemed to have over them. It appears that Gaines, who died only a few years ago, took the worry and the mystery of The Phantom with him to his grave. It is a sad and unique example of how a man's autism ensured his being hurt in the worst way.

It is my own theory (you will pardon my straying off the subject of this book) that The Phantom was a Mad Magazine insider, working blindly for a Gaines rival. In other words, he was a person capable of doing what he was told to do against Gaines, perhaps even believing he was participating in an on-going prank. If The Phantom was, indeed, innocent in this way, he never told a soul. It offers some evidence that the Phantom knew what he was doing, if not why.

As a second pet theory, I have wondered if the FBI was responsible, if they had bugged the Mad offices as they did with so many other publications. Mad must have seemed like a haven for radicals and communists; a woman had complained as early as 1959 that Mad Magazine was a communist rag. It is significant that Gaines did succeed in spooking The Phantom away—never again was any attempt made to disrupt or burglarize Gaines' new offices on Madison Avenue. It seemed that, either way, The Phantom (or his boss) decided his work was finished.

The Phantom has consumed a large portion of this chapter for only one reason: the brave and exemplary behavior of Gaines, the autistic-compulsive publisher, in the face of such a horrid scenario. Other than his initial outburst and the false accusation, he acted coolly. He first attempted to have the Phantom injured and captured; when that plan failed he installed state-of-the-art security, and finally moved his offices, not once but twice.

Gaines fought the good fight against someone who was not only more than his match, but also potentially very dangerous. Whether he suspected anyone else, or whether he learned the truth, or whether it truly remained a mystery, is in itself a mystery. If Gaines did learn something about the perpetrator of these disgusting acts, he kept it from his family and friends. He never mentioned it again, according to the record.

Perhaps many of the fears Gaines suffered were accelerated by the sudden accidental death of his father, who was killed in a boating accident while heroically saving the life of a friend's son. Intense or sudden trauma can exacerbate any illness; in the case of Tourette and autistic symptoms, there can be irreversible damage. In the next section, as an extension of both Gaines' symptoms and of phobias, we will see how irrational ideas become attached to fears.

Superstitions, the Cause of the Common Compulsion

Before I begin, I want to thank Tony Attwood for being the first person to mention superstitions in his work on AS. I had mistakenly thought it was my idea all along. Having said that, I shall not hesitate to note that I did this research independently of anyone else's work.

I love my ideas, fixations, rituals and inflexibility. I will admit this. But no, I am not superstitious. Once upon a time I was, but I like the idea of dropping this apparently insignificant detail into this section because it seems clear that superstitions, whatever their origins may be, are a form of compulsion that most people suffer. I'd have to point out that statistically, triskaidekaphobia (fear of the number thirteen, my favorite number) is the most common of all. Strange that a phobia is also the number one superstition.

I think one of the other most common superstitions is that found among smokers: the "lucky" cigarette. When a new pack of cigarettes is opened, one cigarette is taken out and replaced in the pack upside down. It must always be the last cigarette of the pack to be smoked. I have seen too many arguments and bar fights because a non-believer bummed the lucky cigarette from a friend's pack. Once I made this mistake with a buddy—you would think I had taken his grandmother's 200 year old cameo out of that cigarette pack! I believe that such smokers would prefer that their friends steal money from them rather than to have their lucky cigarette touched.

That great master of communication and public speaking, Arch Lustberg, has noted that the fear of public speaking is statistically ranked above the fear of death. I mention all these fears and phobias because they, as with OCD and autism, seem to be at the heart of almost all superstitions—like they seem to be at the heart of OCD- and autistic-induced fears. Perhaps there is an even deeper link than anyone previously suspected. Bill Gaines once said he physically could not sleep unless there was bread in the breadbox and milk in the refrigerator. This was not the fear left over from a deprived childhood, nor was it greed or gluttony. It was just there, irrational, powerful—like a tic. A regularly scheduled tic of fear.

Lucky charms (NOT the cereal), charm bracelets and amulets are of great interest to me. With these we not only see a pattern common to autism, in which the patient will obsessively collect or hoard whatever it is that catches the fancy; we also see here a strong bridge between OCD and more "normal" pursuits. The charm bracelet is reminiscent of Sacks' theory of tic-enshrinement. Attwood has stated that practically all autistic people have collection obsessions, being unable to pass up any addition for the collection. I think most people are this way.

The most common collections, I believe, are collections of lucky charms, which I prefer to call talismanic remembrance amulets. People afflicted with TS/OCD may become obsessed with a particular type of object, and collections will grow from this obsession. But the objects that are collected approach a talismanic quality for most anyone, and the charms represent this elegantly.

To expand on Sacks' enshrinement theory a bit further, I think we have an example of the enshrining of memories: this is the precise function of a charm bracelet. For many people, these palpable memories become charms of good fortune, and this is not far from a certain type of obsessive thinking. His Holiness the Dalai Lama has always had a fascination with watches, Buddhist rosaries and eyeglasses; his collection of rosaries and watches is impressive. Thus even an admired, unworldly spiritual leader shows this collecting aspect.

When I was a practicing Jew, the cantor at my old synagogue told me that he has never met a rabbi who wasn't a rabid yarmulke collector—one of my own favorite collectibles, by the way. Of course we all know at least one person who has a "lucky" object, ranging from rabbits' feet to socks. I know more than one person who cherishes lucky underwear. I don't, but I am partial to purple ones.

Naturally I do share in this obsessing-collecting habit abundantly, but I do not usually attribute "magical" powers to my objects, even my religious items. Some of the items I carry with me at all times are considered lucky, but I use the word as a figure of speech to represent their intense sentimental value. I have my friend's high school class key, a beautiful nickel-plated Mexican police whistle and tiny brass boat steering wheel my mother gave me, and I always carry some "lucky" coins along with an Othello game piece.

The coins I like to carry are usually a fifty-cent piece and a Susan B. Anthony dollar. My collections of files, bow ties, books, hats, rings, canes and eyeglasses are famous, and I continue to collect all varieties of rosaries from all traditions. I am actually best known for my collection of skullcaps from all traditions, one of which I wear daily. When I was little I collected toy cars, marbles of exceptional quality, and comic books. I'd be a millionaire if I had all these things to sell on today's market—but obsessions, and collections, only go so far.

My own particular habits, lucky charms and collections aside, shade imperceptibly into my obsessive compulsive and ritualistic behaviors. They depart radically from common and cheap superstitious belief, but I am convinced they have the same basic origin. They are deeply rooted in the core beliefs of my religion and heritage: meditation, prayer, the power of the mind, spiritual warfare, demons, witches, spell-casting, healing, clairvoyance. Many of my old superstitions, which I eradicated, were almost entirely sui generis.

Mainly they consisted of what psychologists might call "magical thinking": the idea that situations and objects—even people—can be imbued with or impart some sort of supranormal influence or magic powers. Perhaps there is a scientific basis to this concept. I was trained to it as a martial artist, being taught that anything is mentally possible and that the things a martial artist handles in training are imbued with "magical" powers. Martial arts secrets themselves are seen as magic and mystical charms against evil. Curiously, it is from Buddhism that this martial arts attitude is derived.

The link such common beliefs have with certain schizophrenic delusions is very strong, though it must be emphasized that no relationship exists with schizophrenia or schizophrenic behavior. I prefer you to think of it in a practical sense: because my memory can play tricks on me and I have been known to be absentminded, I have developed certain quasi-superstitious routines, not to be confused with pure OCD symptomology. These are routines that help me remember—they are purely mnemonic and are rigorous on a sliding scale according to their real importance. It suggests that perhaps common superstitions originated as mnemonic devices; I believe OCD, TS and autism show a very distorted or exaggerated instinct of that type.

It is of significance for me to consider what sort of "energy" is "charged" into particular objects. The clearest example I can give you is not one of my own, but of someone who was once close to me: the superstition of one of my grade school friends. Every Friday night, before beginning his weekend homework, my friend would throw all his pencils out the door of his room, sending them flying down the stairs. This he absolutely had to do while seated at his desk, just before he started his homework—and out would come a fresh pack of pencils.

"That way," he said to me, "all of the week's mistakes go with them, down the stairs. I'm free of those mistakes, at least for the following week." Then of course I had my own similar attitudes toward the martial arts weapons I trained with, especially the katana, the Japanese samurai sword. Interestingly, all the Japanese of yesteryear imbued their swords with the same magical thinking.

This pal of mine never used the same pencils from one week to the next, and he never wavered from his perfect GPA. He had no noteworthy disabilities or conditions; anyway, almost everyone I have ever known entertains great varieties of superstitions. My grandmother, aunt and mother would never throw anything away—our house is filled to its nooks and crannies with old keys, wallets, all sorts of tchotchkes. They had a particular aversion to throwing away old keys, though this may have been a Sephardic Jewish custom.

Superstition in one form or another is a universal affliction, and I believe it to also be a valuable link to understanding the function of memory as well as obsessive compulsive behavior. It may even lead us to discover exactly how memory and right-brain thought processes work, and how these processes can be debilitated or destroyed.

Just as certain TS, AS and OCD characteristics may help the sufferer through life, I believe superstitions serve that exact purpose for every one of us. Superstitious rituals, specifically, can help us face life, find answers, put things in order, and get some comfort. These are the ultimate goals we all share. Through these types of superstitions, the normal person can come to see the ever-so-slight refraction of what life is like with Tourette, autism, and OCD. A superstitious ritual might be compared to the flashlight or security blanket some people keep in the bedroom.

For others, superstitions may be somewhat like a roadmap of confusing terrain. Still others actually see superstitious rituals, especially old, established ones, as links to the "other side." Now try to see these comparisons from a tourettic, obsessive compulsive or autistic point of view. Instead of superstitions, there are symptoms and characteristic mechanisms used to deal with those symptoms.

Many times there is a staggering combination of both. These approximate superstitious thinking in a way. From this angle, isn't it easy to experience just a bit of what it's like to handle these neurological diseases? In a sense, superstitions have a religious appeal minus the religion. To me that kind of thinking ultimately tracks us in another apropos direction…

The Paranormal

The possession of clairvoyant gifts is manifested strongly, and is a tradition, in my family, due to our Sephardic Jewish heritage which emphasizes Kabbalah, and the Chinese Zen side. In its literal meaning, clairvoyance is "clear sight." While not having any real connection to compulsive or superstitious thinking, belief in clairvoyance does fall a bit into the shade of superstition. Here I merely wish to bring to your attention that countless Tourette sufferers have reported strong clairvoyant abilities. Every diagnosed adult I've personally met has broached the subject, speaking of clairvoyance from personal experience; such clairvoyance is also reported among autistic savants.

At this point one wonders: are we entering an unexplored region of brain function that might provide us with some practical answers, a region that is unused or ignored? Could it be this very fact that is partially responsible for so many people misunderstanding the nature of Tourette Disease, autism and the other conditions? These questions remain to be answered, but I suspect that the nature of the TS-OCD-autism continuum makes the sufferer hypersensitive to the environment in a way perhaps equaled or superceded only by animals.

I suppose that the hippocampus, involved as it is with memory and the linear processing of memories, might be involved here. I've come to think of clairvoyance as a sort of "readout" our brains give us after chewing on subconscious and conscious facts—something like probability results with some imaginative forecasting mixed into them. In the end we have before us mental information arrived at by way of processes that would put a Cray supercomputer to shame. I believe memory plays a vital role in this clairvoyant process; as we read earlier, tics can manifest themselves in the form of "enshrined" memories.

What if this region is forced to develop its otherwise unused strengths, to help counteract the tic disturbance? Or what if the tic disturbances themselves cause the brain to activate this region by way of compensation, or merely through continual use? This is a fantastic field of possible study, yet I fear no one will ever take it seriously. Remember those folks who think of Tourette Disease as a fantasy? Imagine what they think of clairvoyance....

Dyslephenomena: What It Feels Like To Be Dyslexic and "Dyslalic"

Why nobody's don't wanna do what I ask 'em to do?!

-Thelonious Monk to his producer, demanding to know why no one listened to his suggestions

I've coined the term dyslalia to define the "verbal form" of dyslexia. I'm sure that a certain amount of it occurs with most people when they are tired or drunk, but it happens constantly to many learning disabled individuals. You may recognize "dyslalia" as a spoonerism, which is the mixing up of the initial letters of words in a phrase, such as saying "clack brow" instead of "black crow." There are other occurrences which TS patients experience, such as reversing words or unintentional, unconscious word associations (this is not a tic, though uncontrolled word associating out loud is a common tic)—such as saying "map" when wishing to say "road." There are no known terms for this spectrum of speech difficulties, but a nurse I spoke to recently expressed the opinion that they might be forms of expressive aphasia, or dysphasia.

The root word aphasia is defined as the inability to express words, mainly due to a sort of blockage that prevents the person from either remembering or being able to speak a particular word. It doesn't affect comprehension in any way. Aphasia generally manifests in stroke victims, and I believe it very likely that the same portion of the brain affected by aphasia is affected in TS and other developmental disabilities. Remember the "blocking" vocal tic? Probably the same thing. At the same time, I don't believe dyslalia is the same as dysphasia or aphasia, simply because in dyslalia one actually does say something, and that something at least approximates what was meant to be said.

Numbers are likewise. I often speak them in wrong order, or else say something nonsensical in place of a number. A big problem I have is comprehending the date and the time in one brief glance. Long ago I developed a tic of constantly looking at my watch, but it was partially because I couldn't immediately tell the time; I had to study my watch. This is so bad that people often make sneering faces at me and say, "Am I BORING you? Left something on the stove? Got someone to see, like the president? WHY DO YOU KEEP LOOKING AT YOUR WATCH?"

The most intriguing thing is the anger my watch-studying always elicits. I know it's rude, but the reactions to it are explosive. It is the same with the date; I forget from one minute to the next what date it is, but I am told that date- and time-telling problems are symptoms of Executive Learning Disorder. This learning disorder impairs organization (terrific... when combined with a compulsion to organize everything). ELD weakens memory for appointments, the time, and dates. It seems tempting to lump this disorder with dyslexia, as they seem to go together. It also again reminds us of the hippocampus and how it might be straining to keep our short-term memory working properly.

This particular disability, ELD, is actually not worth discussing other than to say that if it's a problem, then go out and buy calendars, notebooks, sticky notes, whatever works. (Personally I would not recommend these new memory enhancing drugs that are floating about, but if your doctor says "try it," then do so.) Sometimes my room looks like an Alzheimer patient's, with notes and things hanging all over. My mother once said that she didn't have a sticky note on her forehead with "MOM" emblazoned on it because she was too quick for me to catch! It occurred to me that ELD could be a mild form of autism, a "normal person's" autism, if you like. It's mild, and could have almost any cause, so it is not noteworthy. It could be a simple case of chronic absentmindedness.

The worst part of my dyslexia is word reversal. I don't usually mix up letters when I read, but I flip words around, or read them wrongly. Once I was at a carpet store and saw a sign that said "carpet sale." I thought it said "carps are pale." And I remember too many times when I've almost driven into a post or clear off the road after misreading a sign. In spite of this and the precipitating preoccupations, I have a flawless driving record.

And no, I've never even come close to hitting a pedestrian—though there have been a few pedestrians I regret not having run over. Oddly enough, my reading and speaking in languages other than English is only minimally disturbed (with the exception of Gaelic, which would send anyone running for their trifocals and notepad).

When I am tired, I involuntarily use stupid words in place of normal ones, which also happens to everyone, I suppose. But mine are doozies! I might say to myself in the morning, "Jeez, I wonder which Eiffel Tower I should boggle today," meaning, "I wonder which shirt I should wear." The one incident that really sticks in my memory happened in high school.

Arriving late to my art class, I realized my sketchbook was at home—an inexcusable offense in the eyes of my art teacher. We had to keep a sketchbook diary, and he graded us daily on the work we did in our sketchbooks on the previous evening. Trying to explain myself, I said to him, "Well, it's just that I had so many marbles to juggle."

To which the teacher, whom I love deeply, crisply replied, "Well, it looks as though you've lost a few."

What It Feels Like To Have ADHD

As you've probably guessed, when I was in grade school I was recognized as a fantastically gifted if extremely bizarre pupil, and that evaluation never changed throughout my life. (I'm with Isaac Asimov—why adopt a phony modesty? Besides, I've admitted I am bizarre.) When I was in grade school there was no such term as Attention Deficit Hyperactive Disorder. No one had any clue at that time about any developmental disabilities aside from the crudeness they employed in talking about "retards" and "mongoloids." There was no knowledge of attention deficit syndromes, autism beyond Kanner, Tourette Syndrome or OCD.

It's quite probable that ADHD is incredibly common and always has been. It is not too hard to describe: it's like having a million grams of caffeine, cocaine and any other upper you can think of. End of story. Yet ADHD is nothing trifling. For one thing, I think my ADHD feeds my dyslexic problems as well as certain of my emotional difficulties. I can become intensely emotional and lose control. This seems to me to be due more to ADHD than to Tourette Syndrome, but it could just as well be that both are equally responsible—and the end result could be considered a form of autistic behavior.

Being occupied by twelve things at once and not being able to finish any of them is another lovely aspect of ADHD, and this proceeds from concentration trouble. I can generally handle and finish several projects simultaneously—I am notorious for leaving dozens of books scattered about, reading them all at the same time. It makes me absolutely sick to leave anything undone. Now, if someone engages me in intense conversation for longer than three minutes, I feel as if I will run away, screaming like a banshee.

It is almost physically painful to have to pay attention to a person for even that length of time, though in any other situation not involving people my concentration is scrupulous and laser-like. I've also noted that I can observe people intently—as long as they leave me alone! The hyperactivity is also tough to handle, especially if it decides to strike right before bed, making my TS flare. Naturally, in the company of loved ones, the hyperactivity is not too bad. It is at such times that the Jonathan Winters and Robin Williams in me can come out to play.

There are hundreds of books on the racks these days dealing with Attention Deficit Hyperactive Disorder, and that's why this chapter is so short. The only admonishment I make here, which I always make emphatically, is that if you see symptoms in your child or suspect ADHD (also called ADS, or Attention Deficit Syndrome), get it checked. Do not avoid the issue! One of my family members suffered many years with ADHD. His mother avoided taking him to see a professional for over a year in spite of my continuous insistence.

Subsequently, the poor kid was seriously grieving. He didn't know what made him feel so awful, nor did he have any idea why people seemed to be yelling at him constantly. He just couldn't think straight during school, and he began to exhibit frustrational violence. If he became disillusioned with his progress at the school computers, for example, he'd smash in the screen. Imagine: a tiny, scrawny kid smashing in and destroying a computer screen! When they did go to see a doctor, he was diagnosed immediately. Parents, don't make your children go through this hell. ADHD is a serious condition, whether it is comorbid not.

What It Feels Like To Handle Psychological Symptoms

If you see something terrible
Do not become attached.
If you see something beautiful
Do not become attached.
-Buddhist proverb

It's been written that TS is a disease of disinhibition, that there is no "internal editor." This has been compared to the lack of control demonstrated by infants or toddlers, and children who pediatricians tell us have no internal editor. They do what they do and can't control it. It is admittedly troublesome to think of a mature, intelligent adult behaving in a kind of infantile manner, but it happens with TS.

Mind you, this is not to say it involves typical infantile things like incontinence or spitting up with a smile. This childishness or childlike quality refers to things like inappropriate, antisocial and/or improper behaviors that are not counted among the tics (but then again perhaps they are emotional tics). How many TS patients reading this book can remember being scolded or mocked because of "inappropriate" behavior? My guess is quite a few. The same applies in HFA.

I count among the undifferentiated characteristics and symptoms things such as odd moods, low frustration tolerance, disinhibited social behavior (as Dr. Sacks calls it, "a constant testing of boundaries"), impulsivity and sometimes a clinging dependence on others. These, too, could be manifestations of emotional/internal tics. In fact this could be a meshpoint, at which it's easy to see the links TS has with high function autism.

We have to admit that these features make Tourette's Disease seem especially repulsive. If it seems that way to you, imagine how it feels to us. But in light of this repulsiveness, in fact because of it, it's vital to understand the truly crippling symptoms of TS that don't fit into the conventional TS symptomology (other than that they always appear in TS patients). At the same time it's important to remember that there could be more than simply TS at work; there could be comorbidity.

Nowadays, more and more positive aspects of coping with TS are coming to light, much to everybody's happiness. Aside from myriad personality strengths which we all possess, those who deal with TS patients on a daily basis see the enormous strength and discipline TSers manifest in coping. Anyone with Tourette's Disease can tell you about the stupendous amount of work that goes into daily living and social interaction. In a later section we will look more closely at this discipline. Indeed, we've already looked in depth at its essence.

My culture and my religion both teach that logical emotional control is vital. The passions must be governed by reason; expression must be kept in firm custody. (If you are thinking of Mr. Spock, this is even better.) Perhaps not everyone's cup of ginseng tea, but it has done wonders for me. I wonder if Mr. Spock would actually be envious.... I don't mean that the goal is to eliminate emotion. As Diane Duane wrote about the Vulcan philosophy in her fantastic novel, *Spock's World*, "'passion's mastery' is more accurate."

Instead of being controlled, one is in control. Accepting the emotional, psychological trials and weaknesses of TS, indeed, finding ways to use them to advantage, is the sort of goal we all need. My cultural traditions are more along the lines of, "humans act like humans, not like animals." Either way, it's the same thing: "passion's mastery."

This leads me to point out that a big mistake is being made with diagnoses: doctors are saying that anxiety and depression are the major causes of the Tourette patient's symptoms. They are downplaying or even denying the very nature and existence of Tourette's Disease and its symptoms. These doctors seem to think anxiety and depression really have nothing to do with TS per se, that all troubles would go away if anxiety and depression were treated. I believe such doctors are desperately mistaken.

Would TS not cause an otherwise normal person to totally plunge into anxiety and despair, at least now and then? Don't the symptoms resemble anxiety at its worst? That doesn't mean it is anxiety—though we now understand that anxiety can make TS worse.

Since when does depression or anxiety cause classical Tourette tics? Besides, as I've pointed out, TS can appear to be anxiety or panic disorder as well as causing it, and it's far too often simply misdiagnosed as anxiety. In addition, doctors should seriously acknowledge the Post Traumatic Stress symptoms that without doubt plague all TS patients to some degree. Even though the basic medications used for the treatment of PTS, anxiety, depression and TS might be very much alike, it's the correct diagnosis that is the issue here, not the magic pill that will erase the symptoms.

I was diagnosed with panic disorder while in high school. Well, let me inform you that I have always had nerves of steel, along with the slow gains from my Buddhist and Jewish "emotion training." No one can ever tell me that I am not brave, and I would be hard put to find anyone I know who would agree with the panic diagnosis. But this misdiagnosis of panic disorder illustrates some of the dark and indefinable psychological troubles that TS patients can face. What is truly a miracle is that Tourette Syndrome doesn't cause more anxiety and depression than it does. At the end of the day it is lucky for the doctors that the medications are so similar for treating anxiety and TS that their differences hardly matter anymore.

I have felt that these psychological problems come directly as a result of the various stages of socio-environmental trauma that a Tourette sufferer experiences. Just consider: in toddler years, everything seems normal, even promising. In grade school, BOOM! all hell breaks loose, all at once—or else insidiously like a Chinese water torture. Everyone then wonders what is wrong. The family doesn't know what to make of it all, peers are merciless, physicians and schools are ineffectual and the problems proliferate. Just as I said, people with TS should be treated for Post Traumatic Stress Disorder. It would have done me worlds of good. Let us also not forget the deep influence of emotional tics.

Among all the disturbing psychological features there is one that stands out: what I call my "night fugues." The mental states I describe here are called "hypnopompic" and "hypnogogic," describing the state of mind just prior to falling asleep and the state of mind just prior to awakening. Usually just when I'm falling asleep, I'm suddenly startled awake by the sensation of not recognizing where I am.

Sometimes I don't feel that I am where I am supposed to be at that moment. This sounds bizarre at first, but I have heard many people complain of this awful disorientation. Perhaps because of my lifelong sleep disturbances, I am much more aware of it. The general tendency is for me to actually be a bit conscious when I shouldn't be, and so it seems to me that I'm awake when I'm really at least half asleep. Whatever the case might be, it is just plain horrifying to completely wake up from what seems like a comfy, sound sleep and not know where or even who you are!

This terrifying mental state could be part of the origin of the hallucinations I've suffered: it could be that dreams or dreamlike perceptions can be registered on the conscious mind once the extreme relaxation of near-sleep is reached. Many times upon awakening, I've felt that I haven't slept at all, with only the knowledge of a large chunk of time having whizzed past without my perceiving it. Also, in such states it is common for me to experience profound disturbance caused by all the noise in my mind. It's as if people talking loudly and playing music in another room were keeping me awake. Sometimes my imagination keeps me agitated when I'm trying to sleep, pounding at me with nonsensical phrases, ideas, inventions, music, perseverating thoughts and fears. Some of this nonsense reminds me of the dyslephenomenon; some of it is so good I've used bits of it in this book.

The problem with the night fugues seems related to another symptom I've suffered, which is temporary confusion. This does indeed cause great panic, because there is no earthly reason to become suddenly confused, and then just as suddenly not confused. It seems a bit like having Alzheimer's, albeit very insignificant by comparison. Usually my experience is a simple one: forgetting the name of something, not knowing where I am or why I'm there, or getting lost. I know these things happen to everyone once in a while. But when the confusion hits while I'm driving, I feel like jumping from the car just to pull myself together. A neurologist told me that this, too, could be a manifestation of obsessive thinking, but I don't see how. If anything, these "fugues" and lacunal amnesia might be some kind of temporal lobe disturbance, or perhaps even mental tics of some sort. These characteristics seem common in HFA too.

A terrible mental tic that is hard to overcome is sadness. It's just overwhelming, and has no apparent cause. From the time I was 2 or 3, I would have sudden bouts of sadness, like a lingering nostalgia or terrible longing. Sometimes I would just sit and cry silently; other times I would listen to a sad song and cry even more! It reminds me very much of the terrible crying jags that are seen in autism, especially among the low functioning. Among the high functioning, such bouts of sadness are almost taken for granted. But whether this sadness is a tic or not, it certainly provides for some challenging psychological barriers.

Possibly related to this is what I call the "Quit-Looking-At-Me" syndrome (QLAM). In spite of my dislike of the term "syndrome," it fits here. I have noticed that anybody on the spectra of TS, autism and OCD is susceptible to some sort of aggravated dislike of being looked at, of being observed. There are exceptions: in sharp contrast, for example, is Dr. Morton Duran, who feels a desperate need not only to stare but to be intently stared at. Many autistics loudly express their aversion, not only to being stared, but at other types of privacy invasions. Dr. Sacks' famous autistic patient Jesse Parks will explode in fury if anyone asks her "why" questions.

In the documentary, one of the film crew allows his curiosity to get the better of him, and he asks Jesse why she's looking at a particular thing—a cardinal sin lumped in with "why" questions are "what" questions. Jesse immediately wheels on the person asking the question—she seems to know exactly who it is and where he's standing—and barks furiously at him. She sees these "why" and "what are you…" questions as an invasion of her privacy, evidently, or as a confirmation that people are too closely observing what she considers to be none of their business.

There is a list of characteristics that fit the QLAM Syndrome, and at first glance they would seem to be purely autistic in nature. At their worst, they seem like paranoid delusions. Do not be mistaken, they are not restricted to autism, nor are they paranoid or psychotic in the classic sense. They are, however, psychologically very disruptive. Here they are, in no particular order:

1. A hatred of being looked at or observed.
2. Violent objection to any invasion of privacy and personal space.
3. A feeling that others will "wreck" something if they watch too closely.
4. A dislike of generic human closeness, especially physical.
5. A hatred for invasive questions and actions.
6. Fear of being overexposed, especially to strangers.
7. Fear of becoming too "well known."
8. Fear of others using what they know about us against us.

I have restricted the list to eight, because I feel they are the eight major topics, all clearly interrelated, but you get the idea and can easily plug in any additional characteristics.

Perhaps these feelings are strictly a symptom, that is, a symptom that is often ignored because it is wide-ranging and mostly diffuse. Perhaps it is a manifestation of one's own self-consciousness, one's own fears of the public, which are common to all people. Perhaps (I hate to entertain this guess, but

I'll mention it) these feelings are related to common-and-coarse paranoia in a way. One of my neurologists suggested they are obsessions with people staring, and nothing more.

This guess is totally ruled out because QLAM Syndrome is terribly constant and life-long. Individual obsessions are not. My personal belief is that it is related to the sense of self that results from neurological dysfunction or damage. It is interesting that QLAM is seen after certain common insults to the brain, such as strokes, subdural hematoma, and Alzheimer's Disease. I have a friend who was wounded in the head while in the military. He now suffers from QLAM, and the patrons at the quick-shop gas station where he works usually receive the bulk of his wrath.

Everything in this chapter really seems more than anything closely related to the misprocessing of information seen in the autistic syndromes, most particularly in Asperger's Syndrome. In spite of trying to steer away from classical autistic characteristics, we seem to keep coming back to them.

Such confusing, seemingly psychotic psychological disturbances are almost a hallmark in autism diagnosis, and the very same kinds of disturbances are common to TS and OCD. As you will read in the next chapter, Tourette and Asperger may have been tracking the same disease.

Asperger's Syndrome ("AS" or "Asperger's Autism")

The feeling is like glass... if [anyone touches] me I'll shatter into pieces and disappear. I'm not entirely human, and I have bad circuits in my head!
-Diary entry, 1988

You will recall I mentioned that while in grade school I was for a brief time suspected of being autistic, and you will have certainly noted that I've tied high function autism into the text of this book. I certainly suffer strong autistic features, perhaps as coping and defense mechanisms—autism is supposed to be a separate condition, after all. Or is it? All my problems were so overwhelming and I did not know what they were or what to do. Some people thought I was deliberately behaving bizarrely, being cold, withdrawn, hyperactive, making noises, going into my "black moods" as one of my brothers called it, obsessing and throwing tantrums. I discovered much more about these autistic symptoms only later, when I learned that I have AS.

There is a small list of general overall symptoms which indicate Asperger's mild high functioning autism: social or communication impairment; clumsiness; some kind of overt learning disability; other strange or inappropriate behavior. These symptoms can sometimes be deceptively buried, because Asperger sufferers are often geniuses. In fact I found that in the child prodigies I studied, most appeared to have suffered from Asperger's; a tiny percentage who did not have typical AS had autistic features. Only a few very highly experienced teachers suspected I might have autism back in grade school.

They eventually decided it couldn't be possible. I was too intelligent, sociable and, well... weird, in a fun way! AS symptoms can be difficult to see, and AS was not known until recently. The teachers couldn't see the TS either—it too was almost unknown—so everyone just shrugged and dealt with me as best they could. Yet as we have been discovering just in the last few years, autistics can be superintelligent, superimaginative, friendly, sociable and much more. It has also been noted that its incidence, which was deemed very rare, may in reality be closer to an actual figure of one in fifty!

AS is a category of high function autism; almost everyone accepts this fact today. It is due to AS being taken into account that the autism statistics have radically changed. Even here there is dispute: is AS autism, or is it something else? A few experts disagree, but it must be stated that the majority of the best experts concur that AS is a form of autism. Think of it as autism without most of the usual disabilities, or at most very mild disabilities—at least the doctors generally agree that no treatment is necessary. I disagree with this opinion too.

AS falls into a newly named category called "Crypto Sensitivity Syndrome." I am puzzled by this name, but there it is. I think it was intended as an umbrella classification, stressing a kind of hidden perceptual sensitivity disability that interferes with normal function, thus "cryptosensitivity." It encompasses all autistic-like disorders known formally and collectively as Pervasive Developmental Disorders, with the exception of the classic early infantile autism (Kanner's autism) because Kanner's involves mental retardation and unfathomable autistic symptoms.

The term some doctors now use in place of "autism" for most cases is Pervasive Developmental Disorder, though I'm not too sure whether that should be autism's exact across-the-board classification. As a matter of fact, PDD is used when Kanner's autism is not indicated and Asperger's is not suspected or, as is usually the case, when the doctor doesn't know what Asperger's is. PDD is still the label of preference, but a word of caution: whatever terms and criteria one finds in the doctor's office or the research depends pretty much on the doctor involved.

Note, for example, that PDD is differentiated from PDD-NOS (Pervasive Developmental Disorder Not Otherwise Specified"), which has to be one of the most redundant diagnoses in existence. PDD is never "specified" as of a particular type, so why create a category of PDD that is "not otherwise specified"? It's ridiculous. There is so much uncertainty, so much disagreement, on what the terms should be and what they should mean. As more is learned, better terminology will follow better understanding.

As you've read, the severe autism that society recognizes is called Kanner's autism, or early infantile autism. It is actually very rare and generally involves some significant degree of mental retardation, brain damage, and other physical ailments. The Crypto Sensitivity Syndrome label is the newest effort to flee the shadow of Kanner and integrate all the mild HF forms of autism into one syndrome. The few sources I've seen using the term CSS refer to it as a collection of symptoms "exhibited by autistic continuum persons," meaning anybody who shows any symptoms of autism, especially Asperger sufferers. (And it is for this reason that I heartily disagree with the classification "syndrome." This is a neurological disease, like Tourette's Disease.)

Some experts include schizoid personality disorder in this classification, believing the disorder to be a form of autism rather than an evolution towards schizophrenia as is commonly believed. Asperger's Syndrome as a separate entity did not enter into the medical repertoire until 1982, when Dr. Lorna Wing reintroduced Hans Asperger's work to the world. It is possible that some doctors were leaning toward the CSS label before Asperger was reintroduced. Not until the 1994 DSM-IV was Asperger's Syndrome even listed.

It would behoove us to look at the genesis of the delineation of autism. In the early 1940's, the Vienna-born American doctor Leo Kanner was studying children with autism. They were very low functioning, brain-damaged, ill with various physical ailments, and were profoundly retarded. Just a year later, in 1944, Dr. Hans Asperger, also from Vienna and a pediatrician who felt a special link with HF autistic children, delineated the same condition but in milder forms. He independently chose the same name that Kanner chose: "autism" (in Austrian and German it's "autismus"), which had previously been used to describe specific types of schizophrenic behaviors. Whereas Kanner chose the term to reflect some hitherto unknown form of deep, complicated schizophrenia, Asperger chose it simply as an illustration of the nature of the condition.

Asperger made a very accurate delineation which was ignored in favor of Kanner's less accurate one, all because they chose the same name for their respective discoveries. A good example is that Asperger knew autism, in all its forms, to be a neurological disease. Kanner somehow felt it was psychological, involving environment or upbringing—because he had studied many cases in which he could find no sign of brain damage and retardation was difficult to evaluate in such cases.

The attitude that autism was environmental was powerfully driven into the public consciousness by Dr. Bruno Bettleheim. In his book *The Empty Fortress*, Bettleheim made the case that autism was nothing more than the child's manifestation of the parents' desire for the child to disappear. But of course, we all know our environment does affect our thinking: Bettleheim was in Auschwitz during WWII. What he saw happen to many of the concentration camp victims was what he later came to believe was happening to children with Kanner's autism.

Dr. Asperger was following several children with very mild forms of autism; these children were usually of severely gifted intelligence (which means anything above a mean I.Q. average of 132), talented and socially progressive. Asperger saw in them a terrific potential to contribute to society, to be able to live a good life. He followed these children all the way into their adulthoods. That he chose the name "autism" for the condition, independently of Kanner, is no surprise. "Autism" originally denoted severe withdrawal, emotionlessness, and most other autistic traits, albeit as overtures to full-blown schizophrenia. The original German "autismus" literally means "auto-ism," that is, "auto-isolation" or "auto-preoccupation."

The fact that Asperger followed Kanner very carefully is a surprise, because Asperger could have easily challenged the errors Kanner was making—yet he seemed to have done nothing in this regard. He knew Kanner and he were studying variants of the same condition. He also knew that the "Kanner" view was prevailing; at least he could be consoled that Kanner's autism was specified generally as "Early Infantile Autism." How awful it must have been for Asperger, when he felt himself and his work sinking from the public domain while Kanner undeservedly became a sort of legend.

The strangest thing in the case of Dr. Asperger is how it parallels the case of Dr. Tourette: Dr. Asperger was forgotten, too. His work was ignored, and where he was correct and Kanner was not, naturally the medical community chose Kanner's views. The same was true when Freud had his way with the medical community of his time, to the chagrin of poor Dr. Tourette. Both Tourette and Asperger were eventually accused of being inaccurate or just plain wrong. Both Asperger and Tourette felt special bonds with their patients; both were totally forgotten; and both have been vindicated, but only partially and at immense cost.

Both remain without the attention and recognition they really deserve. If you pick up some of the slightly older books on autism, say late 1980's, you will see no mention of Asperger's name whatsoever. If you flip through any kind of medical book short of a comprehensive neurological text, you will see no mention of either Tourette or Asperger. The same is true of any medical encyclopedia. Now, Freud and Kanner, well…! That's different. Their names are plastered everywhere, like religious icons.

As if this were not enough, consider the parallels in treatment of Tourette's Disease and Asperger's autism patients over the years. Consider the feelings of hopelessness the families suffered, the stupidity of doctors, the anguish in school, the isolation from the rest of the family, the institutionalizations. But in an eerie turn of events, the term Tourette Syndrome actually fell from use because the disease was thought to be so rare. Asperger never even received any real acknowledgement until Dr. Lorna Wing researched his work, ultimately re-introducing him and his studies.

Kanner's autism, on the other hand, gave birth to millions of "experts" who propagated Kanner's name and errors. Another similarity is that all earnest study about both Tourette's Disease and Asperger's Autism proved that the earliest observations and guesses were the most accurate. Tourette and Asperger finally triumphed, even if minimally and a little too late. Meanwhile, Freud and Kanner wreaked havoc—for generations.

The most shattering and disgusting aspect of Asperger's descent into anonymity was that he was considered to be nothing more than a Nazi quack. This is the least-known fact about Asperger—but there he was, working in Vienna with no choices, while Hitler marched along. In the United States, it is probable that specialists who gathered around to cheer Dr. Kanner were simultaneously bashing Dr. Asperger for being a Nazi. Nothing could be further from the truth than Asperger being a Nazi.

Asperger was anti-Nazi, anti-Hitler, revolted, frightened and also cornered. He could do nothing but pray that his life's work would not be destroyed. In the most ironic twist of the 20th century, Asperger's work was in a sense "destroyed," not by Nazis but by Americans. It is only meet and just that an American, Dr. Wing, should have rediscovered Asperger's work and reintroduce it to the world. (Even then, as mentioned, Dr. Wing had the audacity to argue with Asperger's findings. Of course she too has been proven wrong.)

As mentioned in their book *Shadow Syndromes*, Drs. John Raty and Catherine Johnson stated that it was really not until the late eighties that very mild forms of autism were "discovered." Of course this is wrong, since Dr. Hans Asperger had fully delineated the mild forms of autism by 1945. Significantly, during the 1980s American doctors were noticing mild autism in the parents of children who were being treated for EIA, and this (finally!)

opened the doctors' eyes. They began to see the genetic pattern and proof of the existence of a whole mild, high-functioning spectrum of autism.

In fact, they were seeing exactly what Asperger had already delineated in 1944-1945, and prior. Just imagine, they thought to themselves, here we have severely autistic children being brought in by mildly autistic parents! The parents are "normal" enough, obviously successful, functioning more or less normally. At first, this revelation boggled the doctors; they were taught that autism was as solid and horrid as the Iron Curtain, and that it meant life as a walking vegetable in an institution.

This little vignette of a medical discovery points up the vast confusion and plain bone-headedness that has tailed autism for decades. Fortunately for us, not the usual chicanery but true research is finally progressing; some doctors are even beginning to examine for neurological changes which they suspect are present in autistic-spectrum patients. Hopefully, a re-evaluation of diagnostic and classifying criteria is around the corner, and we may soon be peeling back the layers that obscure the cause of TS as well as autism. There is today a great reliance on what Asperger wrote, what Asperger patients themselves are writing (we "Aspies" are all incredibly prolific writers), and what they are telling their doctors. (As to writing, a doctor not long ago joked that excellent and prolific writing skills might have to be included in the list of Asperger symptoms.)

In the spectrum of Asperger's autism symptoms, there are many Tourette-like manifestations to be seen. This is the reason TS and autism researchers have in fact already linked autism with TS in general. Among them are David Comings and, inadvertently, Oliver Sacks (he doesn't seem to have actually caught on yet). Autism and TS are believed to involve the same gene. The chief feature of AS is the sufferer's lack of understanding the feelings, emotions and communications of self and others.

Almost one hundred percent of the symptoms of AS are found equally in TS, ADHD and OCD. Because Asperger's autism is to a certain extent open to interpretation, and has been linked to TS genetically, I believe it is possible that at least some forms of autism may be a natural coping mechanism for TS children, if not a characteristic of the same illness. In any case, Asperger's Syndrome is incontrovertibly autism, and if it is found to be a form of Tourette's Disease (and vice-versa would be the case), the arguments will thankfully end, then and there.

Consider: the Asperger symptoms include varying degrees of social dysfunction, lack of emotional display, very little display of what we could call "normal humanity," or normal human interaction and communication, consuming obsessions and rituals—in short, typical autistic behavior. Can you think of a better way for a child afflicted with TS to cope with life? Of course I postulate that every single symptom we've considered in this book falls on the same continuum. Indeed, during special research, David Comings found that out of a group of six young Asperger's autism patients, three of them grew to develop full-blown Tourette Syndrome while retaining their autism in a full diagnostic sense.

Comings' research makes a compelling argument for the fact that autism and Tourette's Disease are on the same continuum. As for obsessive compulsiveness, I believe it is a mild manifestation of two equal "doses" of TS and AS—which is really funny, it's a redundancy. When we clinically define a severe OCD patient, we are looking at what eerily appears to be a full-blown autistic touretter. However it works, we should pay heed to the words of several experts who are telling us that we can learn alot about each condition by way of the others.

Even as we stand at the cusp of new discoveries in the field, awful mistakes are still being made. Again looking at Shadow Syndromes, we read Drs. Johnson and Raty discussing the disconnectedness, the lack of memory association, that rules the lives of HF autistics. They cite the example of a boy who could name all the parts of his bed except the pillow. To him, the pillow was "ravioli"—a pillow does indeed resemble ravioli, hadn't they noticed that? Stupidly, Drs. Johnson and Raty claim that this clearly shows the boy's disconnectedness; they say he doesn't connect or associate the pillow with the bed. Instead, the good doctors tell us, he simply calls the pillow "ravioli," thinking that it really is ravioli. This is sheer nonsense.

Even in a deeply autistic person, simple connections are made. The boy calls the pillow "ravioli" because of imaginativeness or even playfulness, which is ignored as a possibility because the experts continue to claim that autistics have no imagination. Then again perhaps at the time he was merely hungry and tired of silly tests. Perhaps his favorite thing is ravioli.

Autistics do get hungry and tired of tests, like anyone would! We also see this "dysassociation," this dysfunctional association or malassociation (as opposed to calling it "dissociation") in Tourette Syndrome: the person might see an object and blurt out whatever it brings to mind instead of naming it properly. Early in this book, you will recall, I mentioned this very symptom and how it falls into the learning disability category. Conversely, it could represent a tic of some kind. This mistake in *Shadow Syndromes*, which is actually one of dozens, is a clear example of the distance we have yet to travel on the road of knowledge.

Asperger's Autism, A More Personal Note

This section is slightly distinct from the section on my childhood Tourette troubles; I separate it for the benefit of families who may be dealing only with Asperger's or other forms of autism. This chapter will also be stylistically a bit different from the others: years ago I wrote up three sheets of notes, some copied from my taped dictation. These notes are a kind of rumination, reminiscences of a mild autistic childhood. Rather than working the notes into something more formal, I've decided to just more or less transcribe them. This is probably one of the most autobiographical chapters of this book.

As a toddler, I'd run about our house like a quietly demented archaeologist, exploring, investigating, taking it all in—this is among my earliest memories. Our house is what I call a "shoebox" as opposed to the well known saltbox design; it's very long but narrow. It was built ca. 1922 by a Belgian immigrant named Achiel, whose widow, Lisa, became my "adopted" grandmother. An Italian family lived at the home from the time it was built until the last member of the family living there moved. It remained empty for 7 years. In March of 1966, my family took up residence.

I still cannot escape the history, nor what I perceive as the mystery, of our house. Still vivid in my mind are images of going around our labyrinthine, dungeon-like basement and finding a box of paperbacks. These belonged to one of my siblings. Fascinated by the book covers, I'd spend hours in that damp, dark basement taking the books out, examining the authors, titles, and cover art. Never did I read any of them; sci-fi held no appeal for me at that age.

I marveled at the book and story titles, such as *Dune*, and authors such as Piers Anthony; the experience with the box of books in the basement did influence my later sci-fi tastes. All of this was so fun for me, because I have had a lifelong obsessive love for my house. Its history, the people who lived there before us, how it originally looked, everything—it's kept me spellbound for my entire life. Dealing with people, on the other hand, was a bit different.

I remember feeling very lost whenever I was around other people. My few links were with family members who seemed to me like they were able to read my mind; perhaps there was a "Clever Hans" phenomenon happening there. By this I mean that they may have unconsciously picked up on my movements and symptoms, interpreting them more or less correctly, albeit subconsciously. What upset me most about other people is that I believed I was "in tune" with them, yet clearly I was not.

I was unable to communicate well—I was way out of tune. It seemed that the wrong things always popped out of my mouth, it seemed I always did the wrong thing at the wrong time. It wasn't a question of wanting to be understood, really. I had never cared about this; I only wanted to be able to understand and communicate with others in a better way. I now know that being understood and communicating well is the absolute key to "being in tune" with others.

At that early stage in my childhood I did not notice my tics, but did take notice of the difference between myself and non-autistic others. It was partially because I never thought of myself as a "self" at all, and partially because I never thought I could be different than everyone else. It almost seemed as though I simultaneously felt a sort of nonexistence and a meld with all others. When I thought I wasn't human or felt mechanical, I thought everyone felt the same way.

This illustrates a sort of autistic self-absorption: it isn't selfishness or egotism—indeed, it's the reverse. Perhaps it is simply an example of the autistic person's distorted perception. Autistic people walk in their own universe, very much more so than others. I'm still flabbergasted when "my" universe collides with "The Universe" and all the people in it. Similarly, whenever I cross paths with, say, autistic or Tourettic people, I feel an immediate kinship—one that isn't usually shared by that other person. Again, it illustrates one of those collisions that leave me stunned.

As a child I was very sensitive, in almost every way imaginable, but never really showed emotion. I learned to perform for others, putting on and taking off emotions like so many pairs of glasses. But I could never understand people in a profound way—they might as well have been cartoons. The child prodigy's story was very much mine: I've always noted the autistic features present in child prodigies, whether they be autistic or not.

My parents felt that my stunning savant gifts and unbelievably high I.Q. would help me rise in the world. The sad truth is that long years of applied study and experience were required for me to attain a simple, basic understanding of the world, not by any means comprehensive. It has to be emphasized: this is not to say that I lacked emotions, or that any autistics lack emotions.

Whenever I read that autistics are incapable of returning love, I become furious. Feel and return love, YES. Show it, not always—and here I believe is where the echopersonae fits into the scheme of an autistic child's life, probably as it does for the Tourette child. There is simply no way for us to understand what we are feeling, why we feel it, or how to express it. In TS this could be seen as the normal reaction to the tics and symptoms; in autism, it's the reaction to more than symptoms.

It's a distorted reaction to the self, to others and to life. The same is true, for example, with people who absolutely cannot tell their loved ones how they feel. Such people don't show evidence of autism, developmental disabilities or anything else out of the healthy norm—they just can't seem to understand the feelings well enough to say the words. Very old-fashioned men, for example, are like this.

I have always been passionate, at least internally. Passion is linked to obsessions; I learned to study and mimic others with this passion. Any dialect, any accent, even "double-talk" foreign languages the way Sid Caesar used to do on television—I can do them all. I have never had any doubts about my intellect and talents; some people don't appreciate this trait, but I am not abrasive about it. Yet my thought processes have always been computer-like, analogous, in order to better comprehend what others take for granted in their memory and thought manipulation.

This extension of my passions helped me learn several languages. My thoughts and my memory capability are purely visual (and synesthetic); they are immediate and accurate for the most part. What is bad in my memory usually has to do with human interaction: unresolved conflicts, dates, who people are, their names, personal matters like that. The passion, the obsession, doesn't quite go that far, and so I'm as helpless as an Alzheimer patient when it comes to people in general. All my passions, even my deepest, have to be filtered and processed through this holographic computer I have in my head.

Actually, my skills and abilities, other than the pure number IQ, are really average. But I use them more often, more intensely; I use them every second. Normal people don't use a fraction of this potential, and it has been revealed to me that most people don't think visually. This is something Dr. Grandin has written about expertly and expansively.

Einstein said the same thing of himself: he once said that his thought processes were normal but slow to mature. He said that what others think about in childhood never occurred to him until he was a teen, and that's why he was able to penetrate more deeply into questions about space, time and light. It wasn't genius, Einstein said of himself—it was a type of retardation, brought on by the fact that he had to completely translate his pure visual thoughts for others. Most normal folk don't have to do that.

Einstein and I share something else in common: access to wonderful people in childhood and life-long rich environments. This aided us in becoming more "normal," more acceptable. For me, it was not until after my teens that I was able to assimilate acceptable social behavior. This was actually helped by my attitude toward friendship, which I mentioned earlier; if they could understand me and weren't uncomfortable, then I could be comfortable. Friendship depends on this, at least for me. The people I avoid, the people who repulse me, are those who have no room in their heads for anyone else but themselves.

Such people are the true "classic picture" of the developmentally disabled person, and they're supposed to be the normal ones. It's funny, isn't it? The autistic person, cold, aloof, unemotive, self-absorbed, is as repulsed by people of normal health who share the exact same attributes, as he/she might be repulsed by others who share the condition. Is there a lesson here? I think there is: the autistic person absolutely needs the normalcy, the normal attention, the people from whom things can be learned. This explains the certain revulsion autistics might feel toward other autistics—the same phenomenon we see in people with tourettic symptoms.

Relative to this strange "detached attachment" is the way I handle the death of a loved one. For me, as an autistic person, the experience goes something like this: I love Such-and-So, suddenly Such-and-So isn't there anymore. Even after decades, my loved ones who are gone leave fresh, living memories, fueled by my love for them. The memories are vivid, organic, holographic, real—so death is not as deeply negative or fearful for me. There is no "wound" when someone dies. I think Einstein tried to convey this when he stated that in his heart of hearts he had never "belonged" to any one person, any country, any habits, any philosophy.

He was misunderstood; so when his mother died of cancer and Einstein cried for days, his friends rubbed his nose in it. When my own beloved mother died of cancer in March, 2000, I didn't fare so badly, though I too cried for days. When Einstein lost his temper with his first wife, his friends laughed at him and felt sorry for her. When he wept at the sight of injustice, or tried to help his fellow humans, he was accused of being naïve or stupid. When he tried to strengthen himself after the deaths of his second wife and his beloved sister, people said he was utterly without feelings. How sad is all this misunderstanding, and how common for high function and mildly autistic people.

It is this sad misunderstanding, this "cutting out from the herd" inflicted by the herd itself, that causes such a majority of autistics to think of themselves as machines, as Grandin, Einstein and I did while growing up. It was reflected in my deep interest in my own biological functions and my view that they were "artificial" somehow. It seems that I've always felt that I suffer differently from most people. It's as though I were a "duplicate" human, an android (incidentally, the female term is "gynoid"), left in place of what was supposed to be a human being.

Intellectually, I know very well that I am more human, more normal, than I tend to think. Society's responses to us can make us feel like aliens or droids, and society is very good at alienating individuals. Therapy for autistics, at least for high functioning autistics, can be found in the realization that we autistics are NOT so different after all. This very fact has been a renewing lesson for me, which I can only realize now, as a middle-aged adult.

I spent years trying to fill in the gaps that the Tourette diagnosis left. The autistic symptoms, being mild, almost escaped detection—except that they can really be disruptive, sometimes not so mild. It was difficult for me to hold a job more because of autism than Tourette's Disease. Thus the diagnosis of Asperger's autism was and is very important to me, because it is a firm label—that dreaded label that is supposed to cause so much "damage"—it's concrete, I can study it, look at it, learn about it. I can go to a library, the internet, and to professionals who (hopefully) can give me solid answers to my questions.

The diagnosis is in a way more vital than the diagnosis of TS. Autistics like the concrete, the certain, the apparently unchanging. It is the way we learn best, and it is horrifying to us when a thing is unsure, unexpected, unwarranted, unguaranteed, uncertain, inconstant. I like to joke about this and say I'm "anti-un." I also love to say that being uninformed or misinformed is worse than being chloroformed.

The same is true for TS and OCD: if there's an unknown, a change or a surprise, it is torture. We who are affected by such diseases deserve diagnosis and prognosis. Diagnosis and prognosis are almost to be craved, for the concrete assurance, assistance and information. I know that for me it was a horrid craving that I suffered for too many years. And the doctors who blew me off, saying a diagnosis would create a damaging label… galactic stupidity!

What happened to me as an Asperger patient was alarming but simple. When I found the answer to my mysterious, non-tourettic symptoms and characteristics—again, all on my own and with no help—I had trouble finding an expert who was competent to diagnose it. It was just like it had been with obtaining the TS diagnosis. The diagnosis was vital to me and had become an obsession. One of my doctors had stringently counseled against even trying to obtain the diagnosis; he said it would present me with the "danger of being labeled." In that sense, he himself had confirmed the diagnosis. But I have to ask, WHAT danger? The danger of knowing the truth?

There was the doctor I had been sent to see by my therapist; what a moron that man was. This was the first physician I had consulted about the Asperger's autism diagnosis. He couldn't even pronounce "Asperger" correctly; he argued with me about my I.Q., claiming that past and present tests do not "score that high." Immediately, like the other doctors, he branded me a liar and a fool. Then he dismissed me, saying, "Anyone with autism or Asperger's could not have even driven himself here, much less make an appointment to be diagnosed."! What an expert....

Finally I found the autism expert who was truly an expert, a wonderful doctor. She saw me for about forty-five minutes and afterward had no doubt about the diagnosis of AS. When I described what had happened with the moron, she was not happy, and she made careful note of it in the record—which in itself is a highly unusual action. What followed was that the doctor I had first seen was in some way reprimanded, for his unprofessional and rude treatment of me. This man no longer practices here, and I like to think that my expert physician and I were responsible for giving him the bum's rush.

The second doctor I saw was so very nice, and an expert if ever there was one. I may have mentioned something about her previously—I know I've thanked her in this book—but she is worth mentioning again. Firstly, she dealt mainly with children and teens. She went out on a limb in agreeing to see me, for no other reason than to help me. Then she tested me with every intention of ruling out AS. After that stage, she tested me further to confirm that I really am autistic. Once she finished, she had no doubts about the diagnosis. She spoke with me kindly and took a history, but that was mere distraction. What she wanted was to watch me, to spend time observing me closely. As in all such situations, I was oblivious to what she was doing. Now that is an expert professional.

Afterward, she explained it all to me, and explained it all in proper detail in her three-page diagnosis. The very first thing that captured her attention, she told me, was my refusal to make proper eye contact. This, she said, was consistent with autism and intrigued her from the start. (Of course I did look at her—when she wasn't looking—in order to observe and get to know her. That's why I emphasize her kindness: to this day I can still see her very sweet but very professional smile.)

To this day I cannot stand to look people directly in the eyes ("gaze avoidance"), which is a classic symptom of autism. Although it is not generally known that some autistics don't exhibit this symptom. Well, as for me, I've tried all the different tactics designed for shy people, such as staring at the other person's nose or forehead. I can tell you, it is almost physically painful for me to look into someone's eyes or face for too long, when I can look at them at all. My "scanning" of people takes place either furtively or peripherally—called "peripheral viewing." This means that people are observed and studied out of the sides of the eyes.

As far as I can tell it is due to the pain experienced when looking directly at someone or making eye contact. I know I view peripherally so as not to raise suspicion and initiate eye contact. Whether this eye contact problem is some sort of coping mechanism or a mere symptom, or both, I cannot really say. Maybe it's a type of oculogyric crisis or a way to deal with perceptual disabilities. In the "peripheral viewing," there is no voluntary intent, neither to view people in that way nor to deceive. It just happens, as I said, because it doesn't "hurt." Again, I believe from personal experience that gaze avoidance and peripheral viewing are merely preventive against the "pain" of looking at others.

I have never been helped by the fact that my culture finds excessive eye contact and any kind of emotional display to be extremely distasteful. Our culture insists on the goal of rising from animal chaos to "human reason." Staring people in the eye and showing emotion is like an animal challenge as far as my culture is concerned. I was raised in an atmosphere of Oriental social repression. Hardly anyone in my family says "I love you." It simply isn't done, and to stare someone in the eye means a challenge or argument is imminent. This in spite of our Sephardic Jewish background, and the alleged "Latin passion." Funny how a culture, not to mention a family, can actually encourage autistic behavior, especially in children. However, we know that this happens because chances are high that most of the family will be affected by autistic features.

I have noticed that if someone comes to me with a problem or needs help,

I can look them deeply in the eyes and not even think about it—though I notice that I do have to look away at regular intervals. Especially in an emergency, I show no sign of gaze avoidance or peripheral viewing. Occasionally, it is only later that someone might make a thoughtless remark about my "shifty eyes" or "Morse Code" blinking, if they insist on being tactless. It's also been noticed in my family that deep eye contact is sustained when a serious family discussion or conference is held. In this context, the eye contact reinforces the importance of what's being said. Hooray for the Clan Values.

The one Asperger symptom that originally caught my eye is odd or formal (pedantic) language usage; as a specific example, an American using British as opposed to American speech and spelling. This may, but does not usually, include an English accent. I only recently stopped using British spelling and expressions of speech, to help stop the confusion more than anything else. I do, however, have an excuse: growing up, I read and heard a great deal of British literature and often enjoyed English films and sitcoms. I always thought this habit of using British English was an echophenomenal tic of some sort.

I still almost always speak very formally, except when I am reflecting the accent of the person with whom I am in conversation. Friends and even family have remarked on my vestigial British accent, which I inherited from my grade school speech pathologist tutor. Comings' research emphasizes this complicated overlap of the two diseases—meaning the mimicry found in both TS and autism—and Sacks points to it frequently though unknowingly.

Since name-dropping has been such a gleeful feature of this book, I will have you know that some Asperger experts have created a list of famous autistic or suspected autistic people. Among them are Nikola Tesla, Ludwig Wittgenstein, Norbert Weiner, Stanislav Ulam, Isaac Asimov, Alan Turing, Henry Cavendish, Jacques Cousteau and Bill Gates. I don't think it's a coincidence that these people are prominent in the sciences, math and engineering.

Dr. Sacks' favorite autistic patient, Dr. Temple Grandin, holds a Ph.D. and teaches at Colorado State University in Fort Collins. Her particular obsessions, her autism-driven research, have led to a sort of revolution in both livestock handling and animal husbandry, not to mention her fabulous invention called the "Squeeze Machine." This machine offers the deep, gently squeezing pressure which autistic people seem to need.

Like me, Dr. Grandin has found herself trying to logically research and understand the behavior of "normal" people in order to function well. If this isn't the truly gifted scientist at work, I don't know what is. Indeed, her self-descriptive remark was chosen by Dr. Sacks as the title of one his books, An Anthropologist on Mars. This could describe any of us living within the TS/AS spectrum.

Dr. Grandin developed her own special way of navigating in this incomprehensible world: she developed a complete morality, viz., a set of rules to follow that would guide her on her way. Many autistics do this, and become preoccupied with morality in general.

The Moral High Road: Tourette Syndrome, Autism and Morality

This interesting phenomenon which I call moral preoccupation was actually first noticed in TS. It was noted by top researchers that TS patients have very stringent morals, which seem compulsive. The tendency is to develop simple but strict moral codes which are followed religiously, but though these rules may occasionally be inspired by religious beliefs, they are not religious practices. Developing a code of behavior seems to be inherent in the symptoms themselves.

Interestingly, we have learned from several autistic patients that this personality trait is universal among high functioning autistic. Temple Grandin has written about her list of "sins of the system," transgressions that she will never commit because she knows them to be illogical, unhelpful, awkward, or wrong. Both TS and autism patients have some type of similar list, and can be trusted never to digress from the moral behavior they have established for themselves. In actual fact this characteristic seems to be related to the very common compulsion to make lists.

This is an interesting characteristic which researchers have chalked up to typical inflexibility. Though in TS we tend to see many more religious obsessions and fixations, it is possible that they exist in autism as well, in another form. Samuel Johnson loved making friends, drinking, partying, and could chat for hours, even welcoming prostitutes into his social circle; yet he frequently castigated himself for being too lazy to uphold his self-imposed moral code.

Of course, he maintained this code in the form of a list, not of things he shouldn't do but of things he should. In his journals we find constant reproaches in reference to sleeping late, not getting enough work done, not praying enough, thinking too much about sex, and so on. Johnson's moral code is painfully obvious, and must have been especially painful for him to bear. The list itself, however, has the appearance of a juvenile "to do" list.

Clearly the moral code is partially in response to the obsessions that plague so many autistic and TS patients. Perhaps the code is also a defense mechanism; certainly it is an efficient coping and learning strategy, as Dr. Grandin has written. She knew her code would keep her out of trouble in prep school. Jazz composer Thelonious Monk is another good example: he refused to compromise his music in any way, and was even willing to sacrifice himself and his family for the sake of it. Monk certainly had a list, but he kept it in his head.

As for me, I have a very complex moral code-list that has evolved from Noah's Commandments, Kabbalist Judaism, Catholicism, Taoism and Buddhism, but I borrow from all philosophies and religions. I especially like exotic ways of thinking. It doesn't seem to me that my own morals and ethics are related to my compulsiveness or my dislike of change. It is more like a map, comforting to have as a guide, and I will never digress from it because I'll get lost for sure.

This moral strictness is a subject that I consider well worth studying; this short chapter has not really studied it at depth. Perhaps someone aside from me is studying it now. I don't give it much more than abstract, theoretical thought since it's in my blood (and on paper!), but maybe this characteristic will someday teach us about the thought processes in TS and autism that we don't fully understand yet.

In its own way I believe it to be as varied and complicated as any characteristic can be. Serving each person in a different capacity, exercised in various ways and yet serving a single purpose in each case, the moral code is definitely an answer to the social adjustment problems faced by autistic and Tourettic people.

An Affair of the Mind:
Autism, Intelligence, Learning, Thinking and Potential

How many Einsteins... has the world lost by treating [them] as unwelcome freaks...?

-Amy Wallace, *The Prodigy*

Intellectual life, creativity, productivity: things claimed to be at a standstill where autism is concerned. That assumption is simply wrong. People must put themselves into a broader-view mindframe, a view that accommodates autistic intelligence, creativity and productivity. This must be done in order to help the autistic person grow in these areas, to help the autistic person live a much higher quality of life. It also helps to disabuse the popular idea that autistics are like useless robots, mindless, brainless and senseless.

The senses can dazzle, exhaust, terrorize or be taken from us. To what extent our senses are involved in our survival and thought is too deep to be pondered. Suffice it to say that when we consider animal survival skills, and we consider that we are animals as well, we can get a very good general idea of what our senses mean to us. In autism, there are sensory differences from the norm; there is extreme hypersensitivity and hyposensitivity, most of the time occurring simultaneously.

An autistic person may not feel the brick wall that he likes to head-butt, yet a lightly dripping faucet might pound in his head like a jackhammer. He might not notice or care if his knee is scraped wide open, but would be fit for a straitjacket if his clothes were too stiff or rough. An autistic person can have such a terrible mix of hypo- and hypersensitivity that simple human contact is unbearable, yet hitting and head-butting is acceptable. But make no mistake about it: autistic people are very sensitive, and sensible. In addition, they do have senses!

An autistic person clearly has super sensitive, dulled, distorted and hyper-perfect senses, all at the same time—but they have functioning senses as much as anyone else. Senses in autism probably contribute to the rigidity of behavior, routine, and thought processes; they certainly account for the great and sometimes spooky talents autistic people demonstrate. It appears that the senses are the same matter with autism as with Tourette's Disease. Here we enter the realm of pain sensitivity, which goes with the senses; we can fairly call pain the "sixth" sense. Autism commonly shows extremely high pain tolerance, and there are things that could come close to killing a healthy person that do not affect the autistic as much. As I have mentioned, the little everyday things can cause the autistic person much pain.

Remember that Dr. Asperger noticed the extremely high intelligence common in his autistic patients. No one knows why this is, but it is common. I.Q. tests reveal that autistic children and adults who are not retarded, brain damaged or otherwise deeply disabled often range well into the genius level. There is also the incredibly advanced speech, reading and writing noted in Asperger children, though there is some question about their level of comprehension. I remember reading *A Tale of Two Cities* in kindergarten. I had perfect comprehension of the words, but I couldn't begin to comprehend the book as a work of art, a story or even as a book. Still, how many kindergarten-aged children read at such a level?

It may never be fully understood why Asperger's autism and high intelligence occur together as they do; we must remember that it is not purely a matter of Savant Syndrome. Savant Syndrome is applied strictly to otherwise severely mentally disabled patients. Asperger patients, however, range well into genius level, or a little lower, and exhibit savant skills to boot. Consider intelligence itself, and the synonymous connection too often made between HFA and retardation. We have established that in AS there is no retardation or specific disability.

Think: the exact same number of I.Q. points that separates the retarded from the average person separates the average person from the genius. No, I do not especially hold I.Q. tests in very high esteem, but they are worth something; they are efficient measuring tools. Can we pretend that the genius or near-genius is no genius at all, that such a person somehow "copies" intelligence, or even that such a person is in reality retarded?

As Norm Ledgin points out in his biography of Thomas Jefferson, it was the initially uncomprehending but painstaking studying and copying that shaped Jefferson's brilliant creativity and intelligence. In fact it is Thomas Jefferson who is famous for the maxim about manners: that even the most brutish lout could be at least trained to mimic a gentleman to the satisfaction of society, if that brute had the proper model for training—and that in so doing he would eventually become a real gentleman. Was Jefferson writing from experience? Armed with the full intelligence and creativity of a genius, held back by his autism, was it necessary for this great man to study then ape the simplest thing we all take for granted? Was it necessary for him to learn as an adult how to be more human? What a feat of intelligence and genius indeed!

We must pause here and examine another autistic person, one who is not so famous but should be. William James Sidis, with an I.Q. that has been professionally estimated at between 250 and 300, may well be the most actually documented superintelligent human who ever lived. Sidis' parents, psychiatrists named Boris and Sarah, were immigrant Russian Jews with a penchant for ahead-of-their-time educational ideas. Boris was convinced that geniuses could be manufactured, and when his son William was born, he set out to prove himself right. He needn't have strained; little Billy was fluent in Greek by the age of 4—a birthday gift to his father—with another 3 languages already under his tiny belt. It completely escaped Boris and Sarah to show a bit more affection and understanding to frigid little Billy, though Boris was a very kind taskmaster with very modern ideas.

Amy Wallace biographed Sidis in her excellent 1986 book *The Prodigy*. Sidis was extremely famous in his early life (he was born around the turn of the century), having been publicized as the greatest child prodigy ever. Later articles would lambaste him unfairly, and even Carl Sifakis' poorly written 1983 book, *American Eccentrics*, offers a hideously inaccurate and distorted profile. Wallace makes a very well fleshed-out portrait that reaches out to us from the distant past. Sidis, a Harvard graduate at the age of 14, became so tired and infuriated with the life of a prodigy that he became a timid, private person as a young adult. For the rest of his life, Sidis would live in an Arctic chill of run-down boarding rooms, demeaning clerical jobs, and few friends. He had said that the perfect life was a life away from people.

Sidis could not help himself: he wrote prodigiously, perhaps even more than Isaac Asimov, but published comparatively little. He published two works under his own name and several articles and newsletters under pseudonyms. But if his few close friends got too nosey or asked him the wrong question, Sidis would explode in a childish tantrum, covering his ears with his hands and screaming that he didn't want to hear it. His autism was quite glaring, and naturally his childhood as a prodigy was blamed. Even Wallace takes a somewhat unbalanced view on this matter, not taking into account Sidis' obvious autism.

Sidis was obsessed with living a free life. He wanted to live exactly as he wanted; he would brook no criticism of his absolute freedom and independence. In many ways Sidis was a sort of anti-establishment hippie in the 1920s, and was a leader among conscientious objectors. The most recognition he received was constant criticism about wearing tennis shoes. As such, Sidis championed social reform and should really be recognized as one of our earliest civil rights activists.

Though dimly associated with Socialism, later branded by the FBI as a Communist, Sidis was really the ultimate Democrat at heart. Sidis' position as defendant in a civil rights trial, after his arrest for carrying the red silk banner of a Socialist group, marks a crucial time in early 20th century civil rights. He went as far the Supreme Court—and won. As he later said over and over, "All that, because of a piece of red silk. Red silk!"

Billy Sidis was a prime example of prodigy-manufacturing and exploitation gone regally bad. His name even entered the psychiatric parlance: the Sidis Fallacy argues that pushing and pressuring prodigies will leave them essentially autistic as adults. His father Boris was unable to help him in his adulthood, as he died early in Billy's life. Billy's mother Sarah was so unrelenting and shrewish that Billy would have nothing to do with her ever again. In spite of his autism, Billy knew how to survive and flourish, in his own way, in the face of autism, the hounding press, and former prodigy status.

He knew exactly how to dodge reporters, and would move away, changing jobs, if people found him out; he eventually quit this tactic and settled in his beloved Boston. His chief standing and additional contribution to the modern world was his public transportation transfer collection. Sidis can be fairly called the father of modern collecting. One of his two published books is the famous *Notes on the Collection of Transfers*.

Even in this pursuit Sidis was not left alone. Eventually a transfer-collecting cult grew around Sidis' enthusiasm (but not directly around Sidis, he was too autistic). They were soon divided into two major warring factions. No matter what happened to Sidis, he fought back as bravely as he could, getting more and more brave with time. Even his autism seemed to recede somewhat as he approached middle age. Through it all, Billy maintained his famous and overt autismicities, and his courage never left him.

Alas, no one ever took to studying Sidis in earnest, and he collapsed of a stroke in his forties due to high blood pressure and obesity. Within some days he died, in 1944, of the same brutal condition that had taken his father. After his death, the papers continued to hound him and his enemies were still not sated. In the study of autism especially, it is a pity that more writing by and about Sidis does not exist. His mother, Sarah, who lived to the age of 84, dwelled on the little prodigy she felt she had created—she chose to ignore everything else about him.

Dr. Temple Grandin has been the modern exponent of much that we know about gifted autistic thinking and thought processes. I'd like to add to that, if I can. It is true that autistic thought is extremely visual and imaginative in spite of what experts have said, and very inventive. One has only to consider Thomas Jefferson's house, Monticello, or Einstein's General Theory of Relativity. Because I became involved in writing expressively at an early age, it came to be a tool for communication, much like with Jefferson. The Declaration of Independence stands out as perhaps the greatest and most beautiful written document in history, but Jefferson could hardly bring himself to stammer more than one or two sentences at a time.

My experience has always been more in the direction of great writers, poets and orators. Very early I learned the meaning of excellent, expressive writing and public speaking. Dr. Grandin is correct: it is always a visual learning experience, always a matter of being able to grasp the whole, as a living, organic thing. That, in other words, means at least a rough visual grasp. This also helped me to become a successful scientist.

As an artist, I was always able to give expression to my thought-forms. This is not to be confused with Madame Blavatsky and her Theosophical "thought-forms," nor should it be though to relate to synesthesia. In my art there is always a deeply personal combination of synesthetic, metaphoric, analogous and symbolic expression.

For example, in my portraits of Einstein, I try to convey the feeling of being near him, the ideas he created, and the things he enjoyed—the inner visual aspects. I don't just make a photographic copy. To be able to do this I must rely on the "whole picture" of a genuine, living Einstein, not mere words or photos, and that Einstein is the one that "lives" in my mind. Everything I learn is learned in this way. Without the big picture, there is no learning at all.

Autism touched another, lesser-known man, but an equal to Einstein in almost every way. He was not a physicist, but an engineer. Every time we go to the bank, swipe our bank cards, marvel at microtechnology and megatechnology, every time we think about how our modern world has really improved through technological advances, we must think of Jerome ("Jerry") H. Lemelson. The tall, gaunt, fastidiously dressed old New English gentleman can truly be called the patent king. He held more patents than anyone in the United States—over 500, with 40 more pending during the last year of his life, 1997.

Lemelson made an undisclosed but surely mind-boggling fortune. Though he was not renown for it, Jerry was clearly autistic. He obsessed on nature and everyday things; this is where his boundless ideas originated. He said he simply looked at everything and wondered how it could be made better. He wanted the world to be better and measured the success of an invention by how much improvement it brings.

Jerry invented everything "techno," from every type of useful laser technology to kids' games; he established a foundation for young inventors and established the Jerome Lemelson prize, worth $500,000. Through autism, in spite of autism, because of autism… however you wish to view this amazing prodigy of a man, it is clear that the pictures in his mind have made the world truly worthy of the century in which it now finds itself. A great man was lost when Jerry died at the age (in my opinion too young) of 74. Interestingly, his mental predecessor, Einstein, died at the age of 76.

Einstein wrote that his thought processes involved the invention and combination of symbols and pictures. He seemed to have had some trouble translating those ideas, but did succeed eventually. Though this seems an odd place to mention the subject, I think this aspect of autism ties in with echopersonae, because the intelligent autistic is always looking for a model, one that can be at first copied and understood. Later, though there is some mimicry, it is mostly a matter of assimilating the desired characteristics of the model. In other words there is no mere mimicry or "osmosis"; there is a complete absorption of the person being echopersonaed. And it is all done methodically, scrupulously.

Just as Jefferson wrote about the brute who learns to be a gentleman by mimicry, and Dr. Grandin has written about autistics seeking a "mentor," just as so many professionals have asked whether HF autistic people have role models, so the echopersonae itself becomes an early, crude form of artistic and creative expression for the inexperienced autistic person. Einstein pops up frequently in this book because I echopersonaed him as a teen. It was this that helped me cope with overwhelming social and academic pressures.

It was this that made me an expert in his work and in the field of theoretical physics. It was this that alerted me to my present interest in Zionism, and it was this that caused me to gather the courage to create without fear. Today I feel almost like a member of the Einstein family—and all because I "became" Albert Einstein for a few months. Do not be mistaken about this phenomenon: echopersonae does NOT involve the delusion that one actually is the echoed person. That horrible mental illness involves an ego of the type autistics simply do not have.

On the other side of this coin is method of learning. It has been stated that autistics learn by going from the very specific to the general, and this is accurate. Again, using a personal example, I became deeply fascinated by skullcaps; I began collecting and wearing them. From this obsession I became an expert on the history and modern significance of the skullcap, from the sociological and anthropological points of view. As a Buddhist priest I already knew of the Buddhist version of the religious skullcap. As a "crypto" Jew, I came to learn how the custom of wearing a yarmulke evolved, and about its Constitutional legal significance. I even learned how to make them myself; I am often glimpsed jauntily sporting my own hand-made skullcaps.

Without the initial obsessive interest, I would never have learned or accomplished anything. I could not have been induced to learn about all these things only by rote or picking up a book. I am a bibliophile, so I am not knocking books! All my life I've collected them, devoured them and learned from them. Were it not for books, I think my autism would be worse.

The point is that whatever the autistic person's method of learning and understanding might be, it is a system to be respected, to be utilized by parents and teachers. This is comparable to the TS patient whose coping methods must be absolutely respected. There is an authority in command there, and it is the authority of the individual recognizing limits as well as strengths. If there is a vital, primary lesson here it is that the autistic will learn his way, not someone else's way.

Asperger was adamant about the great potential of his patients. He was certainly not under the illusion that his children would fail in life. Indeed, he followed them well into adulthood and watched them thrive and succeed. His major fear was that his patients, being so different from the norm, would never be left in peace. Perhaps his own desperate situation in Nazi Germany, like Bettelheim's, was a part of his observational theories. Asperger feared the Thousand Year Reich, a world that would not progress, would not expand, to accept the types of people he was studying—and he was correct, prophetic, in this fear. How could he not be, knowing that Hitler was at that moment ordering the extermination of the disabled, the elderly, the Jewish people?

This brings me to the personal aspect of creativity, imagination and intelligence. As I have mentioned in passing, my family came from Mexico. I am the first generation of native-born Americans in my family. I've also noted that my family is Sephardic Jewish. Therefore, I was raised with the Sephardic tradition, whether anyone in the family realized our identity or not. We summered in Mexico every year, in my mother's home town, the grand City of Guadalajara. In Mexico, and especially in Guadalajara, the Spanish Inquisition was once in full swing like anywhere else. Our family must have kept at least a vestigial memory of how they had once been in mortal danger.

Mexico is as diverse and (ideally) as democratic as America. It is also as creative, as imaginative. All Mexicans are automatically creative and imaginative, just as all Americans are. Pay no heed to the moronic stereotypes, to the asinine pigeon-holing. My mother and father were both extremely creative, highly imaginative and productive. Like with many old cultures, not just the Jewish, the older generation of women in the family were illiterate, except for my mother, who had a reading level of about 7th grade. I mention all these things because my parents both exhibited Asperger's traits to a high degree.

My father was an expert carpenter, mechanic and welder. My mother, whose only real job had been with an aviation electronics company in Chicago, was not only an expert in all the "womanly" arts. She was also an expert horticulturist and an absolutely dazzling amateur inventor. Mother was never into the grand scale of things, so she did not invent things like improved machines.

Her skill was reflected by the fact that at the electronics company, she worked on top-secret projects for the government, during the Cold War—and her work remains classified. If anything was needed around the house and didn't exist, mother would invent it. If it cost too much at the store or didn't meet her standards, she would re-invent it.

My mother handed down to me this legacy of thinking creatively on one's feet. She taught me how to cook, sew, repair (anything), study (in spite of the fact that she never had a real opportunity to study)—in short, she taught me everything. I had no trouble catching on, because it was a matter of a more experienced autistic teaching a young, inexperienced one. I always argue that anything can be done, because that was my experience. My mother and I shared imaginative musings, had philosophical conversations, created new things together (one thing my mother should have patented was a new kind of storage box she created—but that is another story).

My father, too, was never without his quick wit and vivid imagination. That's why he loved the work of Jules Verne, and that's why he hated science fiction. I learned from my father never to automatically trust an idea just because it was novel or interesting. He dismissed sci-fi and modern film as "pure fantasy." He could never find any value in it—but I will make note that in addition to Verne, my father loved *Star Trek*!

The old man was a different sort—much more autistic than my mother. He never taught us carpentry, welding, or basic auto mechanics. He did teach us to imagine and execute our own projects, no matter how big or daunting they might seem. He taught me patience, an odd sort of patience, for he never had an ounce of patience for people. For everything else, he was the most patient man on the planet. His mind's eye took in everything, and for an uneducated man he was extremely well educated.

He was so well-read that even his relatives could scarcely believe it—he was always quoting an author or poet, obscure and renown. He was an expert, professional self-taught musician and earned a great deal of money in his day, playing with mariachis or solo. In almost every way, my siblings and I are just like our parents. We are even better—because our parents insisted, like all true masters, that we outstrip them in every way before we could pretend to any personal pride. So we all did.

The weirdest thing about my mother, her brother, my father and some of my siblings, is that all were child prodigies, as I myself was. The prodigies were all autistic in nature, which in some way spooks me when I think of it in terms of my family. Now I know this fact because my mother's mother, my aforementioned beloved grandmother, had also been a child prodigy, and because she told me all the stories. Grandmother's most prodigious feature was her memory, but only for certain things.

As she neared her 100th year of life, her short term memory of course was pretty shot, but there was nothing wrong with her otherwise. She, too, had a very autistic streak: she was very mute most of the time, did not particularly like people one way or the other, detested crowds, was deeply private and very obsessive about the way she did things. I remember my grandma with total affection; as a young mother I know she ruled with an iron hand. She single-handedly raised my mother, my uncle and my aunt. There is nothing more creative and imaginative than a job like that!

Asperger believed in the fact that autistics by necessity have to be creative and original in the way they do things; he could not accept that an autistic should be forced or induced to do things someone else's way. It seems that he was writing about my family. Not that Asperger despaired of his patients' lack of reachability, for the matter was quite the opposite. It was simply a matter of accepting his patients for who they really were. He often complained, indirectly, of the misunderstanding his patients had to endure.

More and more often, Asperger dreamed of an enlightened, understanding world with ample room for autistics, and for everyone else. It is no wonder, as he looked from his patients to the rising Third Reich and Hitler's idea of Utopia.

In the next section we will read about a famous man who suffered from the autism/Tourette combination. He was mocked, ostracized, targeted for abuse, and he fought valiantly against his disabilities. He has indeed become a hero to many, including myself; he himself never doubted that this would happen. He became a super-legend during his lifetime, due in no small part to his incredible nobility and bravery—a repeating motif for those afflicted with TS/autism.

Trinkle Tinkle: Thelonious Sphere Monk

I can't be crazy. They had me in a nut house once and let me go.

A person is a genius just for looking like himself.
-Thelonious Monk

It is 1966. You find yourself at an airport, waiting for a delayed flight. Suddenly you run up against a large man in the middle of the aisle. He's just about six feet tall but looks taller, very large and heavy, a noble black man, gleaming black-on-black. He looks exactly like an Ethiopian Jewish patriarch. His impressive goatee, immaculate clothes and eccentric skullcap mystify and please you. But you are also alarmed at his behavior: he is twirling in circles, his eyes fixed on some far away universe. He stops suddenly, flinging his arm into what looks like a sudden greeting high into the air, stomping his foot and lurching forward.

You may notice that he is smiling, grimacing or simply gritting his teeth. Then he fixes you with a concentrated stare. It's suddenly turned into a frightening situation: this fine, noble man, acting in such a way! What is the matter with him? You see all the other denizens of this airport, staring at him in fear, bewilderment or annoyance, while rushing away quickly. Suddenly he stops what he's doing and he hurries away, either sullen and silent or smiling and sheepish. An enigma wrapped in a riddle—and a real work of art.

That mystical, slightly scary fellow was none other than the famous giant of jazz, Thelonious Sphere Monk. Born Thelius Monk, Jr., in Rocky Mount, North Carolina, in 1917, raised in New York City's San Juan Hill area, he has inspired countless composers and musicians. Single-handedly he changed the face of all music, something that had not truly been done since Bix Beiderbecke changed music in the 1920s. Monk's name itself, along with so much else about him, is shrouded in mystery and legend. His father's name appears to have been Thelius Sphere Monk; the middle name "Sphere" was supposed to have been his great-great-grandfather's first name. Since all the direct male descendants bore "Sphere" as a middle name, Thelius' mother decided to name her son likewise.

There is a legend that his real name was, in fact, Thelonious Sphere: his first name allegedly an impulsive quirk of his mother's, and the birth registry entry misspelled. On Monk's birth certificate, it is clear that there is an attempted correction to the first name. However, it is illegible, and there is no trace of the name Sphere or the initial S. There is actually no mistake. All other documents pertaining to his early life identify him as Thelius, or "Thelious," which spelling appears to be the correction made to the birth certificate. These documents confirm that he was in fact known properly as Thelius Monk, Jr., that is, Thelius Monk II.

To add to the mystery and confusion that surrounds so many Americans of that generation, the ignorance of some biographers has lead many to claim that his "real" name was Thelius Junior Monk. This silly error is perhaps a misunderstanding of older documents that list Monk as "Monk, Thelius Jr." or "Monk, Thelius Junior," either of which is correct filing procedure. Thelonious' only son, a famous drummer who goes by the name T.S. Monk, is named after his father and thus called Junior by family. Equally mysteriously, this Thelonious Monk "Jr.," is legally named Thelonious Sphere Monk III.

Moving to the San Juan Hill area in New York City when Thelonious was still an infant, the Monks experienced some racial troubles—from other blacks. The San Juan Hill neighborhood was well known as the West Indian Quarter; West Indians frowned on "ordinary" American blacks. The West Indians would not even refer to themselves as "black," reserving that as a contemptuous descriptor for American blacks descended from slaves.

My father is mostly descended from West Indians, and has always expressed some contempt for "the blacks," even though he is unmistakably black (and Sephardic Jewish, though I believe there's evidence that his ancestors were Falashas, Ethiopian Jews). The Monks had to face this odd, empty racism over and over throughout their lives. Many American blacks were actually hounded by the West Indians, and were prevented from enjoying even simple friendship with their West Indian brethren. It is very fresh in my memory the way both my parents forbade us from fraternizing with blacks.

Anyway, Thelonious Monk established himself at an early age as the purest of pure musical geniuses, and this made him much more acceptable to the West Indians. His mother raised him to be a proper Southern gentleman, and he taught himself piano, both stride and gospel-style, well enough to begin performing publicly by age 11. He sure-footedly learned from the jazz masters of his age, most especially from Eubie Blake, who even in his 90s was still performing. Monk's early musical years are, like so much else, shrouded in the mists of myth and legend: Monk attended Julliard; Monk studied under so-and-so the famous Julliard professor; Monk was thoroughly trained in every facet of music.

None of these rumors has been proved, though it seems Monk obtained as much formal education as he could, by visiting some kind of music teacher who had been trained at Julliard. A friend once hinted that Monk, if he wanted to, could perfectly perform any classical music at will. Of this last rumor I have no doubt; Monk showed consistent brilliance and competence in all facets of music.

After playing the organ in church, at tent revivals and accompanying choirs, Monk blasted onto the jazz scene and re-invented everything. He was recognized, by a few in the know, as the Debussy of the era. Monk inspired and continues to inspire musicians, composers, artists and even film makers, like no one before or since. Strangely, Monk was too modern even for jazz fans of his time; his records and gigs were unpopular. Although more highly respected in Europe, he was misunderstood from the very first.

Monk's friends feared for him more than anything. His devoted wife, Nellie, had to be mother, friend, nursemaid, wife and therapist—though Monk spoke almost as little to her as he did to anyone else. He seems to have suffered equally from autism and Tourette Disease, which drove him to the brink of madness. To this day, no one has managed to really and finally determine what was the matter with him, but the evidence we have gathered offers some clarity.

When he passed away in 1982 at the age of sixty-five (he had been in a coma for about 12 days after a cerebral hemorrhage), even his family appeared to be in the dark about his troubles. Today someone sometimes mentions Tourette's, but it is left at that. A close friend recently made reference to "this Tourette's thing Monk had." Long after his death, Monk's intense privacy has continuously been protected by his friends and family. No one today, however, is in the dark about his genius and influence.

My personal theory, purely opinion of course, is that Monk's main trouble may have been syphilis; he was of the generation of black men who were deliberately infected by the government, in an experiment designed to observe the long-term effects of the illness untreated. This experiment began in the late 1940s. Just a few years ago, then-President William Jefferson Clinton officially apologized to the last known living victim of this horrid Nazi-like experiment.

Prior to that time, no one realized that this terrible thing had been done to so many innocent men. Considering the Monk family's desperate secretiveness, considering that the only authorized information about his condition is that he was neither schizophrenic, psychotic, drug addicted nor manic depressive, it is clear that syphilis may well have been the awful secret, the shameful diagnosis.

I further suspect that Monk lived for many years, perhaps decades, without realizing his situation. One cannot even begin to imagine the pain of those "lucky" few who may have been diagnosed, without ever knowing how in the world they caught the illness. It beggars the imagination to think of the tens of thousands who did not ever receive a diagnosis. A sad, shameful and disgusting end for a great, often mistreated man; all of humanity must feel shame and anger over this. It is no wonder that Monk's family refused ever to discuss details about his symptoms, and that they denied biographers permission to access his medical records.

Sometime in the last decade of his life, around 1972, Monk quit music for good. Although he made a few appearances from '72-'76 , he stopped composing, playing, everything. He never explained why, but a friend has said that it was due simply to extreme ill health and depression. The last few photos of Monk, rarely seen publicly, clearly show a steady deterioration. In 1980, for example, he was photographed looking bloated and tired. In one of the photos he stands in ghastly contrast to his older brother Thomas, who presents a gleaming picture of youthful health. Only a short time after those family photos were taken, new photos show Monk looking thin, frail and very ill.

The Baroness Nika de Köenigswarter recalled that Monk told her he was "seriously ill," and never spoke another word about it. There is a slight possibility that in addition to other woes, Monk may have been suffering the after-effects of two strokes. He may have been afflicted by some sort of demyelination—possibly even a form of multiple sclerosis. Such purely physical symptoms, of course, could result from a syphilitic infection. Some of Monk's friends, such as saxophonist Charlie Rouse, have guessed that Monk was simply fed up and ready to quit the scene. This remark is to be expected from his inner circle, who may have been in on the terrible secret of Monk's true condition. Monk himself coldly halted the question in its tracks once and for all by stating, "I've said all I have to say."

Happily, the world of today can see, appreciate and honor the memory of Monk. In Clint Eastwood's excellently produced 1997 documentary, "Thelonious Monk: Straight No Chaser," there is lots of fantastic footage of Monk. We get to see him backstage, performing, with his wife Nellie, in hotels, at airports. The "true story" vignette I sketched at the beginning of this chapter is a scene right out of some footage. It is a stunning film to watch, seeing the adulation and love that many people showed him.

Equally heartbreaking is watching him trying to stay grounded, trying to keep connected with those around him, furiously fighting his Tourettic and autistic tendencies. We see him gesticulating backstage; we see him twirling and lunging in an airport lobby with several people staring at him in disbelief; we see him in turns surly, withdrawn and dazed or twirling placidly onstage. Contrary to popular belief, this twirling was not Monk's way of directing the band. Monk was a stunning illustration of the fuzzy line between autism and Tourette Syndrome—Tourette experts have seen in Monk the "classic" TS case. Autism experts have seen in him the "classic" Asperger case.

Teo Macero, Monk's producer at Columbia Records and himself a sufferer of TS, features prominently in one scene. Monk, waiting at the recording studio, sees Macero enter. As Macero enters, both he and Monk perform a virtually identical lunging tic at the same time, greeting each other in the true fashion of fellow Tourette sufferers. (Dr. Sacks was greeted the same way when he first met TS sufferer Dr. Morton Duran.) This is a touching scene, as Macero continues to tic his way through the studio as though swimming in a pool, greeting the other musicians as Monk looks on affectionately. Importantly, Macero suffered no autistic features, and this difference between the two men seems to have afforded Monk an intimate link with his environment whenever he worked with Macero. It is also noticeable in this film clip that Macero is the only person with whom Monk feels comfortable in sharing his emotions.

In any case, at certain points in the film it's very clear to see that Monk is frightened, confused and disgusted with himself. In interview, his son T.S. talks sadly about the eventual (I would say inevitable) psychotic breaks experienced by his father. Inexplicably, these episodes are seen in autism but not in Tourette Syndrome, and certainly they are the case with cerebro-spinal syphilis. I do not think the Asperger "psychotic" breaks are necessarily classically "psychotic" in nature. The four episodes I have suffered in my life did have the external appearance of psychosis, purely because there was a degree of dementia, fugue states, and amnesia.

When one considers this as being heaped on top of the usual back-breaking symptomology, of course the whole episode will appear to be psychotic in nature. But I believe it is vital to state with some surety that these episodes are NOT psychosis of any type. They seem to represent a deep autistic relapse and subsequent reaction to the relapse. For example, T.S. vividly recalls his father suffering from extreme insomnia, agitation, lacunal amnesia and dementia, during which times he was incapable of recognizing T.S. or even Nellie. At such times he was clearly immersed deeply in autism, and this was mistaken for dementia and psychosis. Finally, we must also remember to take into consideration the effects of a very possible case of advanced cerebro-spinal syphilis.

The Eastwood documentary, and the story of Monk's life, is a delightful, insightful, and frightening glimpse into the worlds of jazz, Tourette and autism—and the world of racism. It shows more clearly than anything how an individual can suffer for a whole lifetime full of fear, confusion, depression, and anger, totally helpless and alone. Even one of his album titles, "Thelonious Alone in San Francisco," is more chilling than whimsical. Though his wife Nellie said of him that she never knew anyone who could withdraw and concentrate as intently as he did (always said of Einstein as well), Monk without doubt suffered unspeakable agonies. A common tic shown by Monk is his violent flinging of cigarette butts, a symptom that seems to encapsulate all his rage, frustration and sadness.

There is a clip in the Eastwood film, early television video footage of an appearance Monk made on a late night program. Practically mummified in the overcoat he usually refused to remove, like Lt. Columbo, and hidden beneath a porkpie hat and sunglasses, Monk looks for all the world like a hip but homeless windshield-washing bum. Only in the close-ups of him performing do we clearly see his expensive wardrobe, splendid wristwatch, and two dazzling rings adorning his fine, long, slender hands. He performs a number of tunes, most notably his sad, eccentric, angular rendition of "I'm Just A Gigolo."

During the performance of this piece, Monk tics his elbow, shoulder and neck violently between notes; he darts his elbow high into the air while evidently deciding which bunch of keys he will expertly strike next. He suspends his hands almost against his will before poking them forcefully into the keyboard. Upon finishing the piece, he starts suddenly away from the piano, his hands jerkily suspended in the air in front of him. He looks somewhat like a young Stevie Wonder at this moment, with the pose of his hands reminiscent of the famous informal portrait of Samuel Johnson as painted by Joshua Reynolds.

Monk could always think and act in a startlingly logical way. Very early in life he chose to dress in the finest clothing and other accessories. He felt that he could put off the prejudice of others, and "protect his genius," by dressing better than anyone else. Rarely was he seen, even as a teenager, outside of his tightly wrapped overcoat and hat—but beneath these he wore the most elegant suits and ties.

As to racism, Monk often said that after some black friend had convinced him that all white people were evil, that they were all anti-black, he would discover on his own that this simply wasn't true. Monk was impatient with himself for believing racial myths, and went out of his way to ignore the color of people's skin. In typical autistic fashion, all his life he generously and naïvely assumed that others would always show him the same courtesy; of course, they didn't. The government and law enforcement officials were especially brutal to Monk.

Another tic (or set of tics) Monk suffered, which Dr. Sacks often mentions at length in his writings, is the engaging in dangerous or risky behavior. Though this tic faded as Monk grew older, it was evidently a prominent part of his younger years. Dr. Sacks calls this flirting with peril a "testing of boundaries." Saxophonist Steve Lacy tells of witnessing this frightening symptom, and his narrative presents classic TS symptoms: "Thelonious... [had] a love of play... even playing with death... in between sets we would be on the street, in front of the club, and [he] would be playing with the passing cars and traffic lights, like a matador with the bulls." Many people afflicted with TS can relate to this horrifying tendency, and those afflicted with autism also show a failure to understand fear or the rudiments of personal safety.

T.S. Monk says that his father could never have survived without Nellie; Charlie Rouse has suggested that Thelonious might not have even eaten without Nellie to care for him. At such times when autism overwhelmed Thelonious, his Tourette symptoms were in abeyance. Strangely, it seems as if autism sometimes banishes Tourette symptoms temporarily. For example,

Monk would become completely mute and behave autistically; when he was suffering more from Tourette troubles, there was no shutting him up. This lead his son to believe he was a manic depressive—which he was not.

Monk suffered from severe TS symptoms, especially when upset or angry. In spite of the typical social ineptitude, lack of communication skills, and fear of foreign environments typical of autism, which Monk showed in abundance, he had Nellie, plus the brighter aspects of Tourette Syndrome, to buoy him.

Nellie said of him: "Thelonious had continuous nonsense in his head... joking [and] teasing... We had so much fun." Still we mustn't forget the other side of Tourette's Disease. Monk's most important biographer, Thomas Fitterling, wrote,

> *After turning circles [in public] Monk might freeze altogether, fixing bewildered observers with a stare. Slowly the rigid stare would soften to his usual, distinctive look... [The] effect derived in part from a slight squint, and the peculiar expression of Monk's mouth.... This look would then dissolve into a happy beam...*

Monk was ridiculed for many decades because of his tics, which heavily influenced his piano technique. He slapped or stabbed at the keys holding his slim hands perfectly flat, used the piano very percussively, and sometimes hit the piano purely due to his tics: he would bang clusters of keys with his elbow or deliberately hit all the "wrong" adjacent keys while playing. Monk dismissed this tic by saying that only his elbow could hit all the notes he required at such moments.

Captain Beefheart, a musician and pop composer with quite a cult following, witnessed one of Monk's most startling performances. The grand piano, sitting alone while the musicians improvised, had a beautiful vase with roses on top of it. Monk appeared suddenly, almost magically, jabbed out a single note, dumped the entire vase into the piano and then slammed its lid shut. After this he calmly walked off—like the Zen master who blew a single note on his bamboo flute.

Beefheart says it was the whole action, the whole sound, that Monk wanted to achieve. No typical note would suffice; the dropped vase hitting the strings and the slammed lid were necessary. This behavior is a classic textbook example of a complex impulse-tic combination. On the other hand, it is also a classic textbook instance of autistic social impropriety—Monk might have done it out of anger or simply to be funny.

This is reminiscent of family recollections. Thelonious' fantastic but subtle sense of humor was indomitable. Thelonious' brother Thomas was a New York City police officer. Thomas was Thelonious' hero, and all of Thomas' sons adored their Uncle Thelonious. Thomas' wife always kept a large decorative bowl of plastic fruit on the main table of their apartment. Thelonious would wait until they were all at home, then barge in without a word, select a piece of the plastic fruit from the bowl and leave. He would immediately return, saying, "Something's wrong with your fruit, man." He would then stalk back out the door. It always put the whole family in stitches. In the Eastwood film, Monk argues with producer Teo Macero. Although Teo can't see Thelonious, Thelonious is arguing, scratching his head and adjusting his fake glasses—all the while giving Macero the finger.

While his musicians soloed, Monk would rise and dance, twirling around the piano or the musicians while flailing his elbows, and quite a few audiences laughed at him in scorn. In another scene from the film he twirls backstage; when he finishes, he remarks to no one in particular, "I usually do that in the street. Anyone else do that [sic] they'll put 'em in a strait jacket." Then he says, sadly, "People say, 'Oh, that's Thelonious Monk. He's crazy!'" Then, almost immediately, Monk loses all perception of his surroundings and fixates on one of his rings, carefully examining and adjusting it.

Many of these peculiarities affect high functioning autistic people; if confronted, the autistic person might show defiance, ignorance, nonchalance, "absence" or all of these. Monk always did. "Let 'em laugh," he would say when his friends told him that audiences and musicians were mocking him. "They need something to laugh at."

Monk was famous for his high moral fiber and his special feelings about the world. A friend said that "Monk thought he owned the best car, lived in the best apartment, in the best city of the best nation in the world." His blessed naïveté often belied his otherworldly, cosmopolitan aura. Acquaintances and even strangers recognized him on the street during his walks, and even strangers greeted him by name. Monk was affectionate in his own bizarre way, greeting and talking to everyone. His friends were always deeply concerned—Monk had been arrested twice, on one occasion being beaten by the police—and they feared that one day an officer might actually shoot Monk because of his appearance, tics and autistic behavior.

Monk often lapsed into deep silence when upset, and nothing upsets officers more when they want information. In the case of the arrest when

Monk was beaten, all he had done was stop at a restaurant and ask for a glass of water. The era of segregation was in full swing, so Monk was refused, but he would not leave; he stood his ground, unblinking and unmoving. The arresting officer battered Monk's hands, but Monk would not satisfy racism and refused to act or say a word in his own defense. In fact it is said that Monk's hands were struck repeatedly because he was holding on to the car for security and wouldn't let go.

Monk was also famous for his daredevil antics, his adventure-seeking, boundary-testing proclivities and subtle taunts. These are pronounced symptoms of both autism and Tourette Disease—characteristics that police officers really hate. Incidentally, this side of Monk's personality is responsible for the myth that he and Miles Davis once got into a fistfight. It is further stated that Davis won the fight. As a friend laughingly said, "That would never happen. And of course, if it did, Monk would have knocked Miles several miles away!"

Monk was never a pushover. As I mentioned, he had the typical high moral makeup of most intelligent autistics and he had the courage to back it up. If he felt he was right, and usually he was, he simply would not surrender to the wrong view. He was extremely tenacious and was abnormally strong. Monk used to tell his friends about the time he was out for his walk and was attacked by a large German Shepherd.

The beast got firm hold of Monk's right arm; Monk "lifted the dog off the ground and stared him down." The animal was so frightened it ran off, leaving Monk wounded but relieved. As with most autistics, Monk was relatively impervious to severe pain, and in due time the wound healed perfectly. So much for the beating the police gave him—though that event frightened and scarred Monk more than the German Shepherd ever could have.

The eccentricity and individuality seen in intelligent autistics made Monk famous. In keeping with his flawless, flashy taste in clothes, he favored exotic hats. His favorite hat for performing onstage was a black silk Chinese skullcap, of which he owned three. With his long goatee, skullcap, sunglasses and impressive demeanor (which is also common to autistics), he earned the well deserved nickname, "High Priest of Be-Bop." As a youth, Monk pioneered the beatnik tradition of goatee, ascot, sunglasses and black béret.

The instant someone decided to copy him, he changed his habits. Nearing middle age, he became more set in his ways and by then no one dared to try copying him, but simply stole from him. His strong, noble qualities made him a very puzzling, mysterious fellow; his size and tics made him frightening to many who did not know him. It was for these reasons, too, that friends feared the police might shoot Monk, and it was because of his silent but powerful charisma that many people—including the police—harassed, mocked and avoided him.

What is generally not known is that autistics can pursue an obsession for years. Monk's obsession was his music. Autistics will just as suddenly drop the obsession, never to pay it any heed again. This is most likely what Monk did, even before his severe symptoms slowly began finishing him. Charlie Rouse stated that he had asked Monk three separate times why Monk had quit playing. "He never gave me a reason," Rouse stated in interview. At the time Monk gave up music completely, he retired from all society and even abandoned his beloved fancy clothes and crazy hats. He had watched while others stole his glory, saddened by the chintzy change in the foundations he had laid. Even then he was ever the Sphinx.

His creation, Be-Bop, was being commercialized, turning into the big band and soundtrack music of the 1950s and '60s. Monk must have been terribly disappointed and disgusted, watching from the wings without so much as a thank you. It was his work, his vision and his music that became the cool signature soundtrack of the 20th and 21st centuries. The Rat Pack lived and breathed by the musical legacy that Monk created. Toward the end of his life, Monk, unlike the Rat Packers, was like a sad, grizzled, down-at-the-heels Jamaican bum. It was rumored that his spirit had finally been broken. Perhaps it had been. Or, perhaps his body finally quit him.

Even with all the compelling symptoms of Monk's autism and Tourette's Disease, there are other considerations. Monk often presented very slurred speech, a terrible time-lapse delay in his actions and demeanor, and other odd symptoms reminiscent of dementia or brain damage. At other times he appeared to be in the opposite state—and this is when his tics were in full force. This is what has lead me to my second pet theory about Monk having relapsing Multiple Sclerosis.

We must consider that there was the horrid event when someone slipped LSD into Monk's soda pop, which happened sometime in the late 1960's and which friends claimed had permanently affected him. There was the infamous beating the police gave Monk, possibly striking him in the head—he certainly suffered more than one police beating. There is also some evidence, though nothing solid, that Monk may have suffered at least two strokes, and perhaps multiple TIA's ("silent" stroke). It seems that his friends were aware of at least one stroke-like attack.

Monk may actually have been diagnosed with Tourette Disease—it has certainly been referenced albeit vaguely by his former colleagues. Monk was hospitalized several times. If Monk was diagnosed correctly, he may have been prescribed a small dose of Haldol, Thorazine or Stelazine to control his tics. There would have been no other course of treatment available to him in the 1960s. He was known to have seen two of the finest psychiatrists then practicing in New York—one or both of them may have spotted Monk's obvious tics.

It is said Monk had a private therapist, though this could have been in reference to a psychiatrist. The Eastwood film shows evidence of the side effects of anti-psychotic medications, though these effects could have been caused by almost anything, even allergies. Possibly all these facts comprise the secret that Monk's family has always kept. Still, I'd like to delve again into the other possibility, which I suspect is the truth.

Sometime around 1989, the remains of the great composer Robert Schumann were disinterred. It was decided that an exam should be carried out, to see if there was evidence of which grave illness it was that had turned Schumann into a madman as he approached middle age. This was one of the great questions in the history of composers, because Schumann ultimately died of this illness. Many historians had agreed with the speculation that he was manic depressive or schizophrenic, but that somehow didn't jibe with the known facts.

Schumann had become very silent in his middle age, almost totally mute. He suffered from what appears to have been tinnitus, the same condition that afflicted Beethoven. He had become panic stricken, heard voices and saw angels. Unlike Schumann, Monk was not an easily frightened man—but who knows what went on in his mind. Schumann tried to commit suicide by drowning himself in the Rhône, but was pulled out in the nick of time. All he wanted, he later managed to stammer, was to be free of his terrific suffering.

There is an eerie "family" resemblance in the jagged, angular, eccentric sense of rhythm that Monk and Schumann shared. Schumann has been hailed as the true inventor of modern jazz, with his taught syncopation and weird but beautiful percussive dissonance. Late in life, Schumann had become strangely bloated and heavy, like Thelonious. He had been strikingly handsome, almost model material, during more than the first half of his life—like Thelonious.

The 20th century examiners found startling results in Schumann's remains: he had suffered from cerebro-spinal syphilis, which is the most horrid and painful form of the disease. This I truly believe was also the case with Thelonious Monk.

Monk was most certainly infected by the government experiments, which were supposed to have occurred from the late 1940s until the late 1960s. The experiment was mainly carried out in New England, especially around New York and Maryland. Most of the symptoms fit, although fortunately for us, Monk never seemed to have contemplated or attempted suicide as Schumann often did. Not enough were the double racism, the Tourette and Asperger symptoms, the beatings by the police, the public's dumb indifference, the stealing of his work, and the LSD in his soda pop.

No—Monk also had to be struck down by a most monstrous and unimaginable crime, perpetrated by our own government. It is so horrid that perhaps his family went not into deep secrecy but deep denial. What is most vital about my theory is that if it is true, Monk's family is entitled to compensation by the U.S. government—as are so many others. President Bill Clinton awarded monetary compensation to the aforementioned black gentleman from Washington, D.C., who was the last surviving guinea pig of the revolting syphilis tests. This gentleman was born roughly ten years after Thelonious and had also lived in New York City most of his life, fitting the profile of the typical victim.

One is immediately and deeply struck by the fact that this great genius deserved so much more from life. When I first saw the Eastwood film, I was trembling with excitement; I've been a fan and student of Thelonious Monk for decades, and all this footage had been lost since 1968. I had never even heard of it, much less seen it. I had seen a few photos of Monk, but he always looked like someone different in each one.

The moment all the films were discovered, Eastwood decided that a biographical documentary of Monk had to be made. It was and remains a fitting tribute to this giant of a man. After I finished watching this richly deserved film tribute, I was also angry and upset. Monk didn't have to go through all that suffering, he should never have suffered as he did. That is exactly why I've written this book—and I suspect that is the reason Eastwood made his film.

At least today we can comfort ourselves as much as we are able with the knowledge that Thelonious is in a better place—even if that place is only in Eastwood's film and in our hearts.

The Monk In Me

I had suffered other odd problems in the past, which came to mind as I watched the film about Monk. (Luckily I was never infected by any venereal diseases.) Between the ages of twelve and fifteen I suffered a period of quasi-hallucinations, and I was astounded years later to read about how quite a number of people with TS go through this. These are not true hallucinations but perceptual or sensory distortions.

Most commonly I saw rapidly moving peripheral shapes or shadows, and once I thought a ground hog had gotten into the house. I could have sworn I saw it dive under the couch as I was lying there watching television, and my reaction startled my parents, who leapt as high as I did. My mother also suffered from this perceptual symptom: she would often say that she thought she saw shadows moving past her when she was home alone.

My troubles could have been due to sleep deprivation, as sleep disorders of all kinds are found in autism and TS; also there are the half-asleep states. On the other hand, some of the hallucinating or sense distortion might have been related to the dissociative coping mechanisms, or to the autism. I often hear music playing in my head as though it were coming from an external source, but I can never remember it well enough to write it down or play it.

It's perfectly evident to me that these things emanate from my mind; I have no sensation that I'm experiencing genuine sensory input, as does the hallucinating patient suffering from mental illness. Autism provides a more solid answer, though I can't say for certain: the super-sensitivity in autistic people often provides the illusion of a hallucination, but it is none other than the distortion of perception, or the perception of different stimuli that normal people cannot perceive, or filter out.

My sleep troubles consist mostly of scalding nightmares and night terrors, which are basically complex tics leading to panic reactions during sleep. Yet no firm link has ever been made between TS/autism and true hallucinations; they are not considered part of the symptomology. Almost all the personal accounts of TS and autism that I've encountered have mentioned some period of sensory distortion or pseudo-hallucination.

Perhaps hallucinations like these are no more than a symptom of the TS-related trauma, or autistic sensory sensitivity, but there does seem to be a link of sorts: people with autism experience something like hallucinations, but these again are really sensory processing problems. They know these things are not real, unlike psychotic people—and the same kinds of processing problems exist in TS.

I also faced alcoholism, as many TS patients and some high function autistics do, and certainly I held the rank of town drunk during this time. (As Dylan Thomas used to say of himself, "they called me the human beer barrel.") This was a way of self-medicating, and it's no coincidence that I found the strength to stop drinking soon after being diagnosed with Tourette Disease. But I believe it was also a manifestation of autistic obsessiveness—I was obsessed with the pleasure of getting drunk. When you have several conditions and strong feelings knotting together inside you, disaster can easily follow. It certainly did for me: on the average, I would get drunk at least twice a week for five solid years.

Monk probably faced troubles such as the above, and he was known to enjoy his drink as much as his food. There seems to be a link between the sleep trouble, pseudo-hallucinations, sensory distortions, and creativity of an extreme type. It's as if the creativity were a kind of tonic for the troubles, in a directly effective way; not just the uncontrolled creative streak seen in TS and autism, or savant skills, but a sort of drive. And not a drive like a compulsion or impulse control trouble, but simply a drive. Monk was clearly driven, and evidence exists that this drive ran itself down near the end of his career. Though he appeared ill, perhaps he was finally at peace in some way, a peace he would never find in his music.

We all search for peace; we all want it, crave it, and need it. I'm not referring to silly sociopolitical global notions, but to personal, internal peace. The Tourette's Disease patient, the autistic, the Obsessive Compulsive, are most especially susceptible to this urgent desire for inner peace. It is a major part of the symptomology that afflicted persons physically and mentally require peace, require freedom from stress, as much as food and sleep are required.

My train of thought seems to be wandering, but it is not. Something about these neurological diseases seems to be beckoning us to learn more about inner peace, viz., giving ourselves breathing space, time to rest and relax, have fun, enjoy life more. There is something in these diseases (this disease?) that prevents the sufferer from ever finding that peace.

Whether it's Monk jabbing at his piano or Bill Gaines fussing over *Mad Magazine*, the peace just isn't attainable.

Yet there is one man, a Tourettic autistic scientist, who did attain this peace....

The Greatest Brain There Ever Was: *Albert Einstein's Mild Autism*

Chris, owner of Einstein's favorite Princeton, New Jersey diner: "Professor, if the universe has an end to it like you say, what's it like?"

Einstein, laughing: "Not to worry, Chris, you don't go out there!"

-Conversation witnessed by a diner patron in the early 1950s

Albert Einstein is recognized even in countries where nothing and no one else Western are recognized. He is revered as the greatest scientist who ever lived, the man who single-handedly founded 20th and 21st century physics, quantum mechanics, and cosmology. It is rightly said that one Einstein equation is worth volumes of philosophy and metaphysics. Einstein is less known, but nonetheless outstanding, as an expert inventor, having held patents on a special refrigeration system and a new type of camera. In an indirect sense, Einstein also invented the maser and the laser.

He is called the "smartest human being who ever lived." Albert Einstein, with an I.Q. "guesstimated" at around 195, also showed clear evidence of mild autism and Tourette's Disease. In this section we will address several major autistic features Einstein manifested; you will be surprised to learn that these textbook-classic Asperger's autism features are a big part of his fame.

Every child's birth seems marked by an unforgettable event, an event of 'synchronicity' as Carl Jung might term it. The big event reported at Einstein's birth was his grandmother's alarmed exclamation about little Albert's head. "Viel zu dick! Viel zu dick!," she exclaimed ("It's too big! It's too big!"). In spite of what might have appeared to be a case of hydrocephaly, Einstein seems to have been about average in gradeschool; I think too much is made of both his late first words and his "dullness." In fact, his surviving report cards show excellent marks all around, contrary to the "scattering" (wide difference in capabilities) that he is alleged to have suffered.

Later in life, he admitted to being a very slow thinker, a person who needed to immerse himself fully into something before he could hope to comprehend it. He made it clear that he had been this way since his childhood, and he also explained that he often took far too long to answer questions, when he bothered answering at all. Not all Asperger's children show these characteristics, and it is a mistake to hunt for them, or read too much into them if present in a child. In general, this type of behavior will be manifested in the child's unwillingness to point out things of interest to others.

Einstein's parents were lapsed Jews, but that didn't stop young Albert from composing religious hymns on the way to gradeschool. Even then he demonstrated a typical, stubborn independence of thought, though he would become an atheist at the age of 12, after deeply studying then discovering contradictions in the Torah. His taste for order and logic either overrode or blended with his own desires, as is common with autistics of above average intelligence.

He had no friends other than his little sister Maria ("Maya"), nor did he want any. He had family, admirers and acquaintances he trusted—and these he kept a little closer than others. Many "friends" have written and spoken intimately about him—but as he himself said, he never kept anyone or anything close to his heart. "I'm a tough nut [to crack]," he once said deprecatingly.

For the first several years of his life, Einstein was thought to be retarded by a few narrow-minded fools. His schoolwork consistently proved otherwise, but his parents and teachers never stopped worrying about this slow, quiet, aloof little boy. It is said that his mother, Pauline, in an effort to train Albert to fend properly for himself, would take him to the center of town (in Ulm, Bavaria, where he was born) and leave him alone there. Albert was in full agreement with this arrangement: it was an exercise in logic and self-support.

He would have to find his own way home. He was about five years old at the time, and he never lost his way. Naturally Einstein had a powerful bond with his mother. This, too, is not uncommon in autism, and when his mother died in 1920 of bone cancer, Einstein cried inconsolably for the first time in his life; he had cared for her and watched her die in agony, listening to her scream in pain. It is significant to note that, upon seeing Einstein crying, one acquaintance remarked tactlessly, "Well, he has feelings after all. He does care about someone!"

Almost all his life, Einstein seemed cold, eschewing affection and sentimentality. He did not seem to care about the slight lack of understanding he demonstrated toward others, though paradoxically he was very compassionate. Toward himself he seemed almost brutal, prompting Bertrand Russell to write of him that personal matters and emotions "never occupied more than odd nooks and crannies in his thoughts." He was set in his routines and, like most autistics, he was impatient at being disturbed by others.

He simply shut them out, though late in life this particular characteristic mellowed, and he assured students and colleagues that they could come to him at any time without fear of disturbing him. But one of his best friends from college wrote that to Einstein, other people "were like furry little creatures," sympathetic, but furry little creatures nonetheless. It was as if Einstein had no concept of what it is to be human, or to understand the feelings of others. This symptom is called "mindblindness," and most intelligent autistics suffer from it to a degree.

It is because of this detachment and feeling of "otherness" that Einstein came to comprehend the human condition, in the same way that Dr. Temple Grandin did. He had to learn what drove others, why they felt what they felt; but he felt no need to follow suit. Through logic and personal observation, he was instantly able to tell what was, for him, appropriate, what was dispensable, and what was unintelligible. When asked why he dressed poorly all the time, he said, "I wasn't born with [fancy clothes]; why should I need them now?"

Once he was mocked by a friend for trying to attend a black tie affair in an old business suit. Einstein said he would go home and get his old white dinner jacket, put it on, and hang a sign on it reading, "THIS COAT HAS JUST BEEN BRUSHED." Once again, Einstein deflected the attention from himself with a hammy joke. His eldest son, Hans Albert, often claimed his father was a "ham" and adored "playing to the gallery." Autistics can present such an appearance, but it is false.

After a supper party, Einstein was asked by the hostess if he would do her the honor of inviting her again. He said, "No." When chided by his wife, Einstein reasoned, "But why should I? There is no reason to have her back. It is unnecessary." As a young man in Berne, Switzerland, Einstein remarked to a friend, after watching people on leisurely walks down in the plaza, "I just don't understand how people can run around down there like that."

Yet he himself was fond of long hikes—one of the many times he almost lost his life was when he slipped and almost went over a cliff in the Swiss Alps. He liked long, solitary walks, during which he would kick at the ground before taking his next step, as though testing his thoughts. Peter Michelmore, a biographer, said Einstein was fond of walking along the Princeton, New Jersey railroad tracks, balancing himself as he went. It is "autistic logic" to say it is silly for people to scramble about a plaza—when they could be enjoying a real walk.

Einstein passed through two major phases in his appearance, and these have direct relation to typical autistic behavior. Through middle age he was always strapped into a three-piece suit, high wing collar and knit tie. His hair was closely and neatly cropped, in a typical Prussian brush cut, and his moustache, contrary to the fashion of the time, was always short—no handlebars for him. This was for two reasons: (1) he had to dress this way to "look proper"; (2) he felt comfort from the unvarying routine, and the physical constriction (compression) of Victorian dress. Asked by an acquaintance why he wasn't wearing any long johns on a chilly day, Einstein replied, "I dress according to the season. It is summer." These characteristics are inarguably autistic traits. This "Victorian professor" look was his first phase.

Just after middle age, Einstein abandoned his crew cut and let his hair and moustache grow wild, though he always bathed meticulously, shaved his face scrupulously and kept the tips of his moustache short. Peter Michelmore tells us that from this time forward, Einstein "gave little care to his hair, teeth or fingernails." After middle age, he abandoned formal dress, with a few forced exceptions as mentioned above.

These things he did for the sake of comfort and convenience, very common to autistics who are famous for sloppy but comfortable dress and quirky, sometimes slipshod hygiene habits. However, it is not true that Einstein wore the same outfit for days on end (he would have if he'd been able to get away with it), nor is it true that he had seven identical outfits for each day of the week. Some TS/autism/OCD sufferers actually do this sort of thing, but not Einstein. He cared only that the clothes met his standard of comfort, and comfort only.

Once Einstein had been given his first sweatshirt, he almost never wore anything else; like most autistics, he had an "allergy" to wool, though he occasionally liked to wear simple cable-knit pullovers. A family friend (possibly an ex-paramour), noticing his desire for simple, comfortable clothing, found a sweatshirt in an Army surplus store and bought it for him.

He was hooked, and his world-famous collection of sweatshirts added to his fame.

His true oddity was his hatred of socks. After 1930, Einstein refused to ever wear them again; when asked, he stated that he couldn't tolerate the socks getting holes in them. In spite of this, and the further elucidation that he didn't want his wife wasting her time mending the socks, we are struck by his uncomfortable choice. Why would he continue to wear his typical lace-up leather shoes, but no socks?

The possible answers, when examined in the context of autism, can be clear or complex. It could be that he really hated holes in his socks. It could be that he found socks to be a waste of time in general, since he liked clothes that were "comfortable and easy to get at," according to a biographer. Perhaps he liked the constriction of his shoes (always tightly laced) on his bare feet, which again illustrates the need for pressure that is common to autistic people. Like many autistics, perhaps his explanation was the only real reason.

His socklessness, I think, was much like Jefferson's need to soak his feet in ice water every morning upon arising. Perhaps it was a combination of all these reasons, plus his oblivious attitude toward pain; he didn't seem to mind his feet being squeezed into the tightly laced shoes, sweating horribly in summer and freezing in winter. When a little girl asked him why he didn't wear socks, warning him that he could catch cold, Einstein said to her, "I'm old enough that if someone tells me to wear socks, I don't have to!" He was even sockless at his swearing-in as a naturalized U.S. citizen.

Einstein showed two very interesting autistic traits that usually went unnoticed: he kept meaningless lists and he hoarded favorite objects. These two characteristics fall into the autistic love for order, and obsession. Like Jefferson and Gaines, Einstein made lists of routine everyday things, such as expenditures, for no reason. Like most autistics, he was always hopeless with money but obsessed about money—its denominations, structure, the very nature of its existence. After he moved to America, he became fascinated by the coinage; but this, as many merchants and bus drivers noted, did not help him in mastering it.

One day a friend watched him emptying his pants pockets, looking for a letter he had received from the Queen of Belgium, another close friend of his. Einstein's friend observed that "the contents of his pockets were that of any schoolboy's." She noted that he had pieces of string, cookie crumbs, and a penknife. This childlike behavior is also typically autistic. Finally he found the letter, and his friend saw that Einstein had made notes on it. She was excited, thinking she had glimpsed some immortal equations. It turned out to be one of his meaningless lists, of his expenditures for that day.

Einstein is famous for his remark that a man only needs a room to stay in, a bed, a table, a sturdy chair, paper and pencil, "and a wastepaper basket for all the mistakes!" Yet for all that, he was never averse to the pleasures of life; comfortable surroundings, excellent food, good cigars, splendid books and various puzzles, toys and gadgets were all his favorites. What he meant by his remark is that we are who we are and have needs; to strain beyond those needs, to covet and to be greedy, is an asinine waste of time. Einstein often liked to fancy himself a lighthouse keeper or cobbler—because he wanted life simple and devoid of people.

Once Einstein uncharacteristically answered a personal question a relative had written to him. Einstein was asked what his favorite things were. Without hesitation he answered: what he cherished most was his violin, his fountain pen, his watch, and his leather jacket—all gifts from loved ones. (The fountain pen and leather jacket, like the sweatshirt, feature prominently in many photographs of Einstein. He loved to stick the pen into the right-hand side of his sweatshirt collar for easy reach. Since childhood, I also had this habit—the number of people remarking on the oddity of it has always struck me.)

He also had a massive collection of the most innovative games and puzzles; Einstein was a nearly unbeatable Go champion, swift as a Zen master, and he also played Dr. John Nash's game, Hex. Needless to say, he had a massive working library with some of the finest and rarest books available.

This habit of placing a high regard on certain objects and always having them close by (hoarding), is an autistic-obsessive trait that reminds us of superstition. Einstein was no superstitious pack rat; the most deeply personal letters written to him have been lost. He didn't cherish or save that sort of thing.

Even the highly revealing love letters he wrote to his first wife, Mileva, were saved only because she took them when she left him. He was absolutely callous about family photos. His one cherished honorary doctorate, one among dozens, was the one he received from the Lincoln College in Nebraska, a black men's college. The rest of them he threw into a corner—he called it his "boasting corner."

It was common for family and associates to notice Einstein's detached and self-stimulating behavior, as well as some tic activity. His favorite behavior was to twirl a lock of his hair while thinking, and he would often rise in the middle of company, as if in a trance, leave without saying a word, and proceed to play his violin. One of Einstein's relatives remarked on the beautiful, childlike image of Einstein standing alone, "tugging" at his hair.

When Einstein and his colleagues got stumped over some problem, Einstein would say, "I will a little tink [think]," then stand up and slowly pace the room, twirling his hair. Then in a few moments he would have the correct solution. His colleagues always expressed the wish to be able to "go with him" on these inner journeys. Many scientists who worked with Einstein have admitted to twirling their hair; as Dr. Banesh Hoffman eloquently states, they did it with the hope that "some of Einstein's magic would rub off on us!" As Hoffman noted with a laugh, "It never did!"

His tics seemed almost randomly scattered, but they were consistent enough. He frequently made rude, childish gestures for no reason, and often stuck out his tongue. The famous photo of Einstein with his tongue sticking out is evidence enough: he was photographed upon leaving the hospital after his gallbladder operation. On the back of the original photo, which was given to him, Einstein wrote, "To the doctor my tummy, to the picture-taker my tongue."

The most evident tic Einstein suffered lead many people to make an erroneous assumption about his face: many people believed Einstein's eyebrows were situated in an unnaturally high position. In fact, this was because of his life-long tic of raising his eyebrows very high when he was in deep thought or mentally absent. Whenever Einstein was angry or relaxed, his eyebrows were quite normal.

In fact, Einstein's expression in later life affected people to a high degree—his face was always very serene, "angelic" coming up often as the adjective of choice to describe it. Simply speaking, Einstein had finally found a comfortable expression to keep on his face—many autistics do this—and rarely expressed any real emotion facially. This, too, is common in autism. The Einstein expression has been famous ever since; not necessarily only in connection with him, but in the world of public speaking. The Einstein expression is taught as the proper, open expression one must use when addressing an audience.

The Einstein expression was even more powerful during Einstein's famous "absences." One of the hallmarks of autism is the "complete absence" of the person, even though the body is present. Though we addressed his self-stimulating behaviors and tics, these are on another plane compared with Einstein's "absences," the ones his colleagues wished they could share. Even in the newsreels, Einstein is captured in close-up, smiling alertly and raptly into the camera; then almost immediately the smile fades and the gaze wanders. Even on film it is palpable that Einstein is "no longer there."

These "absences" are common to all autistics, and featured in Einstein's life so significantly that everyone who knew him wrote something about it. In her excellent biography, Antonina Vallentin gives us a beautiful description of this autistic behavior.

She notes beforehand that Einstein was not the ridiculous absentminded professor type that we all know so well; his attention was rapt and complete for whatever or whoever needed it at the moment. His autistic "absences" were thus very pronounced. Vallentin is worth quoting extensively, because it is perhaps the sharpest vignette anyone could ever write about autism:

> *Once I saw him stir [his tea] with concentrated attention... as if wrapped in a dream. The whirlpool he had produced in [his] cup so completely absorbed him that he did not... hear [anyone] speaking to him.... A separation seemed to take place between his mind and his body... [he] would be there... alive to the simple pleasures of life.... Suddenly he would fall silent and stop listening.... He would rise to his feet without a word, or remain... motionless. He would be unreachable... he would neither see nor hear.... [T]he eclipse... was total. He might appear lost to us for a long time, and then return to us as if he had never realized his absence; he might remain without movement for a time that to us appeared an eternity, or return... rapidly.... [O]ne never quite lost the feeling that his presence among us was only a temporary loan.*

Such words have been written extensively about many autistic people. An implicit note Vallentin makes is of Einstein's laserbeam-like concentration, yet another hallmark of autism. So Einstein, like all other autistics, also fully aimed that beam of concentration at his "absences." Another interesting note: TS/autism people love to watch spinning things, which is reflected in Einstein's obsessively watching the tea being stirred.

Einstein's former son-in-law, Dmitri Marianoff, put it even more eloquently, if more briefly, in his Einstein biography: "I saw [Einstein] transported to an abstract, inaccessible domain; he would stand immobile like a monolith." Marianoff's sentence and Vallentin's sketch were written decades apart.

Not uncharacteristically, Einstein himself censured both Marianoff and

Vallentin precisely because of such privacy-invading comments. Of course Vallentin was in love with Einstein, and that was why she was ultimately made *persona non grata* among the Einstein family. When her book came out in 1954, Einstein himself loudly denounced it, as he had denounced Marianoff's book two decades earlier, accusing them both of being liars and exaggerators.

Marianoff was cut out of the family picture because he had divorced Einstein's stepdaughter, and because he knew Einstein was a skirt-chaser. This is probably Einstein's version of the deep privacy cherished by most autistics; in any case he came from a very private family. What I find truly irritating about Einstein's "absence" characteristic is the way some writers have used it: they claim it as evidence that Einstein was epileptic. Nothing could be further from the truth.

Einstein was ultimately unique and recognized because he was not an overly selfish or cruel person. Autistics rarely are, but even when autistic behavior can seem reprehensible, there are, as we have seen, valid reasons for it. Einstein was also a typical autistic of extraordinary intelligence in another way: he was a peaceful, wise, good, tender-hearted man who suffered with the world. Getting him to admit it was another matter entirely. As a young professor, Einstein had gathered around him a group of admiring students. He treated them, as he did everyone, equally, and as equals to himself.

Even to them he could display prominent autistic habits, such as his habit of refusing to speak to (and glaring at) anyone who had mysteriously "fallen from his graces." Former student and biographer David Reichinstein once found himself on Einstein's "angry list." Reichinstein distracted him with an interesting speculative remark about Martians. Einstein replied, "Why, that is very interesting." As soon as Einstein set to pondering the question, his anger toward the young man vanished forever. This type of distraction tactic is today a much-practiced redirection of autistic behavioral flare-ups.

I can readily identify with this symptom, because I've always had it. Whenever a particular person angers me, I sometimes lapse into a trembling, icy silence that can last all day. Whenever this kind of symptom afflicts me, I notice I become physically ill too. This is certainly a form of the autistic mutism, and it seems that being mute, at one time or other, will always remain part and parcel of the autistic experience.

Dr. Grandin considers Einstein a "cousin" because of the striking autism that accompanied his striking genius. Einstein confessed to being a visual thinker, and always admitted his inability to sustain complicated mathematical activity due to the symbol-juggling. The math symbols were not his symbols; he found this very confusing and hard to bear. Often he would dismiss an erroneous equation by saying, "Ach, that can't be right; he's so ugly!," emphatically pointing to it on the blackboard

Einstein could be a trifle absentminded, but only with regard to people—his memory and attention were excellent otherwise, as many of his biographers have noted. He was thought to be retarded when young precisely because he was very quiet, deliberate, and kept everything to himself. His childhood acquaintances nicknamed him "Biedermeier," which was the name of the clunky Victorian-German furniture of the day. This nickname translates roughly as a person who is slow, ungainly, awkward, naïve, and unaware. Kids today would use the term "clueless."

He himself stated that all his work was based on asking childlike questions. It is significant that Einstein's work concentrates on time. If pain is our sixth sense, as I have asserted, time is certainly our seventh sense. Einstein was insensitive to all kinds of pain, like a typical autistic person, but was deeply sensitive to subtleties like certain types of pain, and time. This in turn gave the basic foundation of Relativity theory. Finally, Einstein suffered, as all autistics do, from severe stomach and bowel trouble, and this was not helped by constant over-exertions at his work in addition to the miserable, poverty-riddled first quarter of his life.

The obsessiveness about sticking to one task indefinitely is another disabling characteristic of autism—it was simultaneously Einstein's blessing and curse. Too much has ultimately been made of what Einstein's actual I.Q. was, because it was acknowledged that he was the most intelligent being who ever lived. Of course he was not—this was simply what the public had labeled him. Certainly it is simple enough to estimate an I.Q. for Einstein, but no one has yet accurately done so.

We are reminded, too, of the interesting fact that Einstein several times almost lost his life, yet would walk away from such situations in an almost robot-like fashion, unfazed. Once he was thrown from his capsized sailboat; his legs were entangled by the sails' ropes and he nearly drowned. When he surfaced, he still had his pipe clenched between his teeth. Einstein almost died twice of physical ailments: first a major heart attack in his fifties, then much later, anemia resulting from a special diet. In his early poverty-stricken early years, he had nearly starved to death. He gave new meaning to the phrase "play through the pain"—as all afflicted persons do every day.

To him these brushes with severe illness, serious accident, and death constituted no more than minor irritations, and like all autistics he loathed the attention they brought. When he finished recovering from his heart attack, he snapped at his wife, "It is past! Let us talk no more about it." All she had done to elicit this remark was to admit she was worried about him.

When he almost fell from the Alps while still a student, he merely said to his friend, "I'm glad you carry that stick around all the time." Einstein showed the typical, terrible self-neglect that borders on thrill-seeking, common to most autistic people. Obviously he was not especially sensitive to, nor afraid of, pain—and his daredevil sailing bordered on the suicidal.

Yet Einstein was also somehow hypersensitive; it is difficult to pinpoint it exactly. He often became angry at certain people for no perceptible reason, and would not or could not explain why. There were environments he could not tolerate—and these idiosyncrasies match autism very well. He was easily moved to tears, but one biographer claimed (apparently baselessly) that all the Einsteins suffered from sensitive tear ducts! The full grown, mature Einstein wept sadly at his mother's death. He was deeply moved by his visits to India and Japan, and he cried openly upon giving his goodbye address to his Japanese hosts. He cried again when he learned that the bombs had been dropped on Japan.

Perhaps one story more clearly illustrates Einstein's environmental sensitivity: he and some acquaintances were traveling together in separate cars, Einstein nestled in the back seat with several others in one of the cars. When they had to pull over for a car emergency, the driver of Einstein's car hit a bump that caused the rear bumper to strike the ground and screech.

To the driver's amazement, he noticed in the rear-view mirror that Einstein's eyes were wide, his face gone white, horror-stricken. When Einstein dismounted, it was very difficult to coax him back into the car again. This from the man who literally laughed in the face of death. Perhaps it was the noise, the feel, or perhaps he hated cars. He never did learn to drive and never attempted it, though he enjoyed going on drives.

There was a flip-side to this coin, as evidenced by a friend who went for a walk with Einstein. Einstein was addicted to tobacco, and very partial to cigars. His friend noticed a frazzled stub Einstein was smoking. It fell from his mouth, and after a few seconds' thought, Einstein picked up the cigar, brushed it off and stuffed it back into his mouth. "But what about the germs?!," his horrified friend asked. "Ach, I don't give a damn about germs." This fascinating disregard for hygiene, which we noted previously, is in stark contrast to Einstein's obsessiveness. Certainly he was not "dirty"—he was fastidious about bathing—though many people wrongly assumed that he was an unclean person.

His addiction to tobacco also demonstrates what could be either typical human frailty or autistic tendency. Although sensitive to liquor (he would not drink wine and regarded beer as poison), tobacco was a part of his diet. When he was forced in old age to suck on a cold pipe and drink only Sanka because of his stomach, his friends saw something like self-pity, for the first time. None of this deterred Einstein, who would ask to sniff his friends' pipe tobacco (perhaps evidence of a sniffing tic). He would steal his office colleagues' cigarettes, shred them into his pipe and smoke them as fast as he could, before anyone caught him.

He demonstrated a classic autistic tic by repeating his own words to himself (palilalia) after he had finished speaking; this lent him an additional air of slowness and oddness. He also demonstrated copropraxic tics in the form of rude gestures; one example, showing Einstein thumbing his nose and sticking out his tongue, has been immortalized in a newsreel. The other immortalized example is the photo of him sticking out his tongue. No wonder: Einstein's term for photographers was lichtaffen, "light-monkey."

He could be very childish and rude in general; it is not for nothing that a close associate called Einstein a "kicker of sacred cows." Once, when he went with some friends to an art lecture, Einstein sat in the front row and heckled the pompous artist-lecturer, whom he had never met. He could be as cruel to himself, often calling himself a "fat pig" or a "worthless old man." Once he said, with no trace of self pity, "It would have been better if I had never been born."

Albert Einstein is to date the most photographed person on the planet, about whom the most has been written. His charismatic, stunning, otherworldly appearance (actually another autistic trait) inspired more writers and photographers than anyone in history. The autistic tic mentioned above, that of raising of his eyebrows, attracted much attention to his beautiful eyes. With his "angelic" expression, Einstein was demonstrating a combination of self-stimulating and tic behaviors, which undoubtedly "helped" him think.

There are plenty of photographs, especially from his youth, that show him furrowing his brow and frowning, a much more common "grimace tic" among people with TS/autism. It is important that more often than not, many photos of Einstein do not show the raised eyebrows and distant gaze, but rather the involuntary sour grimace, penetrating glare and angry brow that is so common to both autistics and touretters. In his final years, as he aged far too rapidly, his expression also changed. He looked, as one friend remarked, as if age and illness had seared away all unnecessary features, leaving only infinite wisdom and sadness. A teenager who met him at the time described him as "angelic."

Another interesting trait which is evident from newsreels is Einstein's rather catlike, feminine, mincing gait. This odd gait, along with the total stillness of his arms while walking, are both actually listed among typical symptoms of Asperger's autism. Many family members and close acquaintances thought Einstein walked this way because he had large, flat feet and varicose veins. One of his friends unkindly wrote that Einstein "paddled along" rather than walking. His doctor thought it might be due to the varicose veins, which troubled Einstein all his life. None of these conjectures is true.

Einstein displayed stiff, awkward body language and a certain degree of clumsiness, which we have already seen is very true to high function autism. Also, in the newsreels his gait appears very delicately studied, which it probably was: it is an example of an autistic person doing his best to fight awkwardness and walk like everyone else.

A Japanese official, commemorating Einstein's visit to Japan, wrote in a very Zen style that "Einstein had a quiet way of walking, as if afraid of frightening away the truth." In the end, he continued to walk in that lightly springy, uniquely autistic manner, without swinging his arms, until old age and illness made him unsteady. After that, he had to walk more normally, to swing his arms and slow down a little, to keep from losing his balance.

As was addressed in a previous section, Einstein, in spite of some clumsy awkwardness, was an expert sailor as well as an avid hiker. People who went sailing with him noticed how he seemed to blend into nature when active, like an old athlete. Many people were amazed at his thick, muscular body and apparent grace. It was the reckless behavior that supplemented and emphasized these other qualities—Einstein was a stubborn, eccentric sailboater. He refused to keep or use life preservers, and would not allow anyone on his boat to wear one.

He was famous for charging directly at other boats, then veering away at the last second, to the great horror of his boat-mates. He would laugh like a little boy and do it over and over, expertly veering at the last possible second. As has been stated so often, this bordered on the suicidal, excepting the fact that it afforded Einstein the most fun of his life. This habit reminds us of Thelonious Monk playing in traffic in New York, dodging oncoming cars. (It also reminds me of J.R.R. Tolkien, another Asperger sufferer, who drove often when younger, but eventually quit. Tolkien would charge down the pedestrian-busy roads in Oxford, gleefully crying, "Charge 'em and they scatter!")

In his later years, Einstein showed two more characteristics, and these are the ones we should think about more than any others. The first characteristic was the appearance of his eyes: they became loaded with sadness. Everyone remarked on this. The second characteristic was his mouth: it had become weighed down with bitterness.

After decades of illness, bereavements, fighting the Nazis, long after his first-born, a daughter named Lisa, was given up for adoption, after his youngest son, Eduard, was institutionalized due to schizophrenia, after his elder son Hans Albert fought with him and turned him away, Einstein had been worn down to the nub. Friends said his Eduard's mental illness struck him most deeply.

After the divorce from his first wife and the death of his second, after the deaths of his mother and his sister, his two most beloved family members, and especially after the bombs were dropped, he had had enough. He managed to remain serene and peaceful, as his close friends noted. This all proves one thing: Einstein was as human as the rest of us, genius or no genius, autism or no autism. We must never forget this.

If autism has a "personality" to it, if it manifests as a particular "type" of person, which seems to be the case, then Einstein is the ideal. Though he displayed tourettic behaviors abundantly, such as obscene gestures and inappropriate behaviors, this is not inconsistent with an intelligent autistic person. While still living in Germany, Einstein attended a huge Nazi lecture which was intended to expose and destroy "Jewish physics." Every time Einstein and his work were attacked, Einstein applauded and cheered loudly. Friends were afraid the Nazis would recognize him and shoot him in the street—shades of Monk's friends and their fears—but he kept at it, oblivious to everything but the stupidity and humor of the situation.

Einstein died in 1954 at the age of 76. It is very significant to notice the last photos of him; he looked like a nonagenarian. His aortic valve was leaking, and would eventually burst, killing him instantly. His only blandly intoned question for the doctor was, "Will it be painful?" No doubt he was more haunted by the memory of the loss of his mother than any real concern for himself.

While he was still at home, before his final illness struck him down, the doctor called because Einstein had felt ill. He was experiencing his typical mixed attacks of heart trouble, stomach pain and irritable bowel syndrome. The doctor stirred a medicine (we do not know what it was) into a glass of water and told Einstein to drink it. This he did—and immediately vomited in the sink. Afterward, Einstein casually handed the glass back to the doctor and said flatly, "Do you feel better now?"

Because of this typical "Einstein behavior," his own doctor proclaimed him to be a "genetic mutation," super-intelligent and incapable of fear. His charisma, his hammy personality, his mental fugues and his colorful eccentricities (actually "autismicities") made for a most fascinating public persona indeed—a nice definition of "personality."

Hans Albert, Einstein's oldest son, often remarked on his father's colorful, show-off attitude, a real "personality." Could there indeed be "personality types" on the spectrum of TS/autism? Our next section will explore this question—and provide an answer.

The Tourette and Autism Personality Theory

If autism is a neurological culture unto itself, who might its historical role models be?... Einstein...?

-Valerie Paradi

Dr. Oliver Sacks is the first (actually I think the only) expert to talk about a "Tourette personality," though Dr. Comings' research also seems to be leaning in that direction. There has also been some quiet speculation about a HFA personality since the publication of Elijah's Cup. In his article "A Surgeon's Life," Dr. Sacks talks about the personality characteristics he noted in many TS patients: a wry, "elfin" sense of humor, a tendency toward pranks and odd associations, lightning wit and reflexes, a certain insouciance, belligerence and argumentativeness, and great creative intelligence shown by prodigious writing, math, musical and artistic skills.

There's more in the "Witty Ticcy Ray" chapter of *The Man Who Mistook His Wife for a Hat*; in it he also mentions competitiveness, significant athletic ability, earthy language and "chutzpah." There is much in the autism literature, first seen and most especially emphasized in Asperger's paper, that makes similar claims about an "autistic personality." Dustin Hoffman's performance as Raymond Babbitt in the 1989 film *Rain Man* immortalized forever the typical (though at best low to mid-functioning) autistic person.

It is in my opinion sad that so many people in the field have mocked this "personality theory," or simply don't care. Some experts have insinuated that Dr. Sacks is no more than a *National Enquirer* pseudo-doctor. One neuropsychiatrist told me, "I don't care about a patient's personality, or any personality nonsense. I'm interested in neurochemistry. Period." Yet it just so happens that I see the "personality" inherent in the neurochemistry, in myself, my family, in every case I personally recognize, and in all the cases I've ever seen or about which I've read.

Dr. Sacks is probably on to something of socio-psychological importance in TS and autism understanding and treatment. As he has written, we've fallen victim to a "soulless neurology and a bodiless psychology." He's looking for a way to re-establish the holistic approach that Dr. Tourette, his two predecessors, and more recently Dr. Asperger, had suggested.

From my own experiences, the best illustration I could give of the TS personality is to compare myself with Jonathan Winters and Robin Williams, as I wrote. During my first year of college, a friend told me I was like a combination of William F. Buckley and Groucho Marx. Before you swear that you'll add me to the list of individuals you never want to meet, let me offer reassurance that this is only true at times. I'm not always like that. No one, as my best friend says in her inadvertently Zen manner, is always anything. But it will give a better impression if I add that this is as involuntary as everything else associated with TS. I wouldn't trade my wit, speed and humor for a cure, but it still doesn't make it voluntary.

The "autistic personality," from my experience anyway, is in line with Einstein's character. There is a great deal of childlike innocence, and that does not change. There is hypersensitivity to certain things and hyposensitivity to others. There is a shy, retiring and privacy-loving quality in the autistic personality, and some of it borders on apparent paranoia. Then again, as I always emphasize, there are lots of open and relatively extroverted autistics. So many characteristics that are the opposite of TS seem to appear in autism, yet as we see, they easily co-exist. In fact, I think they are in symbionce.

Some of this is also developed over time. It was important to the autistic person as well as the Tourette person to methodically learn and rehearse some kind of public persona and that's what I did—many times over. There is no such thing as charisma-in-a-can, but I look for the nearest thing whenever possible. It is a matter of finding the right characteristics, either in others or within myself, then display them.

This personality, if we take it seriously, seems to infer that we probably see more Tourette's Disease and autism than we realize (unless we know nothing about TS/autism, or don't want to know, in which case we never see anything). My guess is that more than a few dozen performers and other public figures have TS. I believe there are as least as many in less public professions who have autism. I think it prudent to leave it up to you to guess who they might be!

In his book, *The Man Who Mistook His Wife for a Hat*, Dr. Sacks makes many cogent points that obliquely refer to the Tourette personality theory. He has written much more extensively about it in his magazine article about the surgeon. He has also made references to the playful, imaginative, creative and "open" life of so many autistics. It really burns me that so many medical professionals have relegated Dr. Sacks' ideas to the realm of cryptoneurology, simply because the research gives inconvenient answers. Shame on you! I know who you are, and I know what you've written!

Dr. Sacks is one of the few in the field courageous enough to say that we need to learn from Dr. Tourette, we need to go back to the good old clinical methods, when doctors listened and learned form their patients instead of offering no more than conveyor-belt treatment. That is no treatment at all. Sacks knows that Dr. Tourette was a good old-fashioned doctor in the noblest sense of the term. We are in sore need of at least a few such doctors today. Doctors should not merchants or peddlers, interested only in the quick and easy dollar. We are not "consumers," neither desirable nor undesirable. We are patients, we are human beings, and we demand real doctors!

The personality idea seems to address the deep fissure that our society has caused to grow between body and mind; doctors ignore too much in their tunnel-vision efforts to treat symptoms. The TS and autism sufferer as a whole person cannot be treated or dismissed in this manner; and remember that we see much more of the same thing happening to autistic patients. In fact, this is the biggest barrier to advancement in learning more about autism. It's as if doctors are simply unwilling to step outside their own minds, even for an instant.

We have what I have called a continuum on which lie probably dozens of diseases. You could think of it as a spectrum on which doctors are only seeing single colors, not the whole rainbow or the light it gives. Imagine—a patient sees a doctor who pronounces, "Yep. He's a purple." Then everyone applauds the doctor's conservative discretion. When doctors come along and say, "We have a rainbow here. There is interplay, and it's all of a piece!", everyone boos them off the stage.

The psychiatrist I saw after I was originally diagnosed with TS was utterly incapable of dealing with the personality or social aspects of the disease. She seemed to be forever conveying the message, "Sorry, I don't do Tourette's. Aren't you feeling even a little bit depressed? Don't you want an antidepressant?" She was comfortable pushing antidepressants and she desperately hoped I would suffer from something she understood, like depression. She was uncomfortable dealing with things she didn't understand, and made no effort to try and understand them. TS and autism have their sufferers in a stranglehold that reaches into the nether regions of the brain and comes spilling out through the personality, covering our bodies, personal space, and environment.

Doctors sometimes behave like someone who goes to a person that's bleeding to death and says, "Oh! I don't really have that much to do with bleeding; how about a back rub while you die?" All anyone can say is that if the TS/autism patient can go out and learn as much as an expert clinician is supposed to know (have no doubts: this happens a lot) why are there so few expert clinicians? If the lay people involved with TS and autism are capable of research and of advancing terrific theories, how come the doctors can't even think straight? There is no excuse!

We must face a fact: the Tourette and autism personality theory would explain quite a bit of our social trials. It is filled with all the right answers. As Einstein said, a good theory "answers everything that's mysterious, and that's what a good theory should do in the simplest possible way." This much is all anyone can desire from a good, working theory. There is too much of the attitude that only the obvious tics or autismicities really matter, and everything else is anxiety, neurosis, whimsy or just plain stubbornness.

Perhaps it's hard to take the TS/autism patient as a whole because it means we have to flex our brains, make more allowances and do more work. Acknowledging the personality theory means you're stuck: not only are there tics and autism to worry about, now there's an entire personality that goes with them! As you'll see in the next chapter, families are particularly suspicious of the personality theory, even while accepting other facets of Tourette's Disease and autism.

More of My Early Years

One of my older sisters took care of me when I was a toddler (she was around eighteen then, I think). She had an almost psychic understanding of me and exercised a patience that could have served Job as an instruction manual. I will always believe that, were it not for her, who knows where I would be now. Ten times worse off, that's for sure. I feel the same for my maternal grandmother. Now that they're both gone—my grandmother passed away and my sister living a remote, xenophobic life in Colorado, in the throes of her own mental problems—I truly miss them every day. I realize that I've always required much special attention and care, which my gramma and my sister gave above and beyond.

My few very pronounced, severe Tourette symptoms began to manifest at around the age of seven. In fact, they were much worse then than now. Prior to that age, I was a very energetic but frail, undersized child. Of course autism manifests around the age of three, unless the child has EIA. In my case it seems to have manifested earlier because I was very precocious. My hyperactivity was constant, so I basically had no rest from it; I think that's mainly what caused me to develop into a prodigy.

This is in contrast to my infancy, when I had an almost ghostly calm, according to my family members. They nicknamed me "Casper" as much for this as for my silence and physical appearance. But later, the Tourette symptoms went unnoticed for a long time because the gradually increasing violence of the tics I suffered were viewed as normal development for me. So much energy, so much intelligence, so much creativity, so much weirdness; why worry?

I remember squeezing my eyes shut constantly, a separate tic from the blinking tic. I was also very hard on my clothing since I would clench a tiny corner of my shirt in my teeth for hours. I had saliva-soaked shirts with little "suck-points" all over them, making me look like a giant wet cocklebur. The collars on every shirt I owned were also pretty battered, as I yanked on them constantly to relieve a constriction I always felt around my neck and throat. Almost all the tics I suffered seemed very self destructive, and I was tempted by obsessions to hurt myself.

This violence expanded, and I developed a tic of destroying library books, along with the impulse to throw away my things. I also have vague memories of hitting myself, but remember them as being motivated by feelings of retaliation against my disobedient, clumsy body. To this day I find that if something's gone wrong or if I've been clumsy, I hit myself as hard as I might strike a mugger in self-defense. These symptoms—are they TS, autism, a combination of both? I'm afraid I don't know any more than anyone else's guess.

Awful, intense emotions shook me. I'm surprised my teachers didn't suspect manic depression. Yet I never really felt I was different in any way as a child, which seems opposite of other TS and autism experiences. Of course, I absolutely hated being a "child" and did not want to be one. My mother always told me I had been born old. I could never understand why I sensed incongruous tension in the people around me, though I do remember always being puzzled by others in general. The only significant difference from others I remember feeling as a child is pain. Never will words be able to describe it, so I call it "pain."

It was so intense that every time my sisters dropped me off for my lone walk in the cemetery (my favorite thing to do at the age of 3), I would beg them to leave me there, in a grave. I believe this was my age of definite TS onset, according to what my sisters can remember. Obviously the autistic tendencies showed much earlier and were totally missed. This is natural—as I keep indicating, when I was little there were no such terms as "Asperger's" or "ADHD." Tourette's Disease was supposed to occur only in one person out of 100,000! Even high function autism was misunderstood, and was confused with Savant Syndrome for many decades.

The worst tic I had, when I was about seven, was squinting at things and bringing them almost into contact with my face in order to look at them. The congenital myopia I suffered, which affects my entire family except my father, didn't help. These tics, along with sitting about five inches from the television, are probably partially responsible for ruining my visual acuity. I've had to wear ever-thickening glasses all my life. (No contact lenses! Eye tics, remember?)

Even though bad eyesight runs in our family, mine is the worst—and I have quite a few bouts of oculogyric crisis every day. Today I'm presbyopic, and I have to wear big, heavy trifocals. One thing I must admit: I love my Ben Franklin (Executive) trifocals. My eyes have never been more comfortable, and I no longer have bad "viewing" habits or tics, other than the usual peripheral viewing, gaze avoidance, rolling, darting and squeezing my eyes shut.

There is something that occurs to me, now that I am thinking about my eyesight and glasses. Long ago I experienced a very painful incident that I'd like to share with you. One of my brothers once told me that it was his opinion that I wanted something to be wrong with me so badly I could "taste it." This happened during a time when my doctors were trying to push me away and I was in utter desperation, seeking the answer to my problems. I speak for every Tourette's Disease and autism sufferer when I tell you: NO, we don't want something to be wrong. When we are undiagnosed, we want something to be done.

We want to know what is wrong—we know something is—and we want it made right. This feeling only gets more powerful after the diagnosis, so don't think the buck stops there. I was reminded of this because my father always resented the trips to the eye doctor so I could get new glasses, always trying to deny the fact that my eyes were poor. See the similarity? Denying a disabled person's pain is like denying new glasses for someone with bad eyesight.

Aside from this, too many people, like my family, believe that the only thing these neurological diseases require in the way of treatment is self-discipline and proper motivation. Such beliefs are offshoots of denying the TS, the autism, and the accompanying personality characteristics. This is not only sad, it's repugnant. When will folks see that people with TS and/or autism are the most disciplined and least frivolous people anywhere? Individuals with disabilities will understand this daily fight; you who fight inner (and outer) demons know exactly what I'm saying. Few others ever fully grasp it.

For those who suffer no disabilities, what a blessing you enjoy! But let me ask you: How well could you handle people mocking you or running away in fear, every day? How would you like being scolded like a child no matter what your age? How well could you handle deeply personal criticism, often from strangers? How would you like being called a liar every time you expressed how you felt? As you are reading this, bear in mind that a Tourette/autism patient can and does handle all this and more, every day, like a seasoned pro. What of the deeply autistic person, who cannot speak out? What other choices are there for us?

Some of the absolute garbage I hear some people say about TS and autism makes me want to turn to violence. At other times I'm so hurt I actually cry. So much for Buddhist detachment. Therefore the onus is really on the professionals, the researchers and experts, the people who take concepts or theories and make them household words.

We as patients can only do so much; this book is about as much as I could manage, and this is precisely my point about the lack of support. How it is that people are incapable of recognizing TS/autism baffles me; the media still represents "crazies" as people who have tics and make gestures… people with autistic tendencies are accused of being "nerds." When will it end?

A Child's Tale

Once there was an unusually pale and mild-tempered baby boy. He never ever cried. He was happy, always in an apparent state of meditation unless he was cooing and gurgling with glee in his own little world. He learned to walk, speak (and swear) fluently before the age of one, and by the age of three he could speak several languages, imitate anyone perfectly, speak dialects and double-talk.

Everyone thought he was superhuman: he had an evident lack of general needs and a detachment that strengthened his family's awe. A stoic little one, never crying when injured and rejecting any special attention to his injuries. You've guessed it: the baby was me. Turns out everyone was wrong, wrong, wrong about the superhuman part! I am now viewed variously as an attention freak, a freak of nature, a mental case (or a genetic mutation—for the better, perhaps?).

I know from personal experience that it's not healthy for anybody to be branded either a prodigy or a pathological weirdo. Usually everyone thought I was long on weird and short on prodigy. No degree of exaggeration exists in the fact that I was viewed as some sort of inhuman life form. Then with the inevitable changes brought on by adolescence, a peak in TS symptoms and school trauma, the perfect little boy became something like the ungodly stepson.

This time period also saw an acceleration into deeper autistic tendencies. It is still shocking and painful to realize how little respect my relatives actually have for me, but this is not all-inclusive. As I've written, a tiny few of my family members are as loving and respectful as is appropriate to our family. I think many kids with TS/autism go through this alienation. I can't see why, really. What do people think they can accomplish by making their kids feel rotten?

School was not so bad, really, but for a few ignorant and cruel teachers, counselors, and administrators. My grade school teachers in general were very supportive in spite of the fact that they truly wondered whether I might be an extraterrestrial or a mutant. It is with complete understanding that I now look back on those years; I was educated in a first-rate grade school that was nonetheless the proverbial one-room schoolhouse. We had two floors, and each grade, K through 6th, had its own room. I really loved it for the most part.

One teacher I do recall with a shudder is the one I had—either 2nd or 3rd grade, I can't recall. She was a monster, and was merciless toward me. Thinking back on her, she seemed like a bitter ex-nun with a biker streak running through her black soul. One of my sisters, the toughest one who is also one of my best friends, finally had to go to the school and threaten to rearrange this teacher's nose. Only then did she stop tormenting me.

It shouldn't surprise you to know that even doctors did not know enough about TS or AS; because TS was considered so rare, and AS was not even known, no one bothered to study. What is so surprising is that looking back, I can see that the teachers for the most part seemed to do the correct things instinctively. That is probably due to the fact that the true statistic for Tourette and autistic symptoms, and the full-blown diseases, are probably close to one out of every one hundred children, according to a study Dr. Comings did in Los Angeles.

Today, experts and teachers accept a Tourette's Disease statistic of one in 5,000. The autism statistics are changing so rapidly, increasing so steadily, that no one may ever finally reach an accurate statistic. Extremists say TS occurs as often as 1 in 50, and autism of some type may exist in as many as 1 in 50 across the board. Today there is a tendency to see through the old inaccurate stats separating males from females.

I had to work with a speech pathologist and another special education teacher. They came to the school once or twice a week, and I remember them with great fondness. It wasn't so much because I was slow (remember, child prodigy) but that the teachers didn't know what else to do. The speech pathologist was a practical necessity: I had a very sibilant "s" and it's still vaguely detectable, as is my Latin accent (which a few people confuse with an Italian, Jewish or French one).

In retrospect, it's possible that the other special ed teacher's job was to erase the last of my Sephardic-Mexican-by-way-of-Chicago accent, though I'm told I never had any kind of accent as a child. I suppose I also had the peculiar speech typical of high-function autism. To be honest, I never knew the reasons for the presence of so many special ed attachés in my grade school education. Why would anyone bother explaining it to a junior ET?

At home, it was another matter. The older I became, the stronger the reprimands grew. Everyone thought my symptoms and behaviors were deliberate. Parent-teacher conferences, when they did occur, were a farce. There were some teachers who had the keenest contempt for me, and an even keener desire to remind me of that fact every three seconds. Also, around this time in my life my siblings were marrying, leaving home.

Then my beloved grandmother and aunt moved back to Chicago for about a decade. In my early childhood, my grandmother and aunt had lived with us; my aunt moved away first, then invited my grandmother to join her. This period, leading into my junior and senior high years, is one of the loneliest I can remember, even though I never really wanted for attention. But don't believe I ever showed my pain. I didn't know how; I didn't know it was "pain."

School Days, School Days:
What I Wish They'd Known In Those Days

Let those who choose to carve a human soul to their own measure be sure that they have a worthy image after which to carve it, and let them know that the power of molding an emerging intellect is a power of death as well as a power of life.

-Norbert Wiener, autistic mathematician and creator of cybernetics, referring to teachers, 1952

Since I've referenced the grade school years, I want to begin this section with a small "ode" to my grade school. Truly, we all learn everything in grade school, because we learn our ethics, our social place, how to study and apply that study, everything. The rest is comprised of mere details. It's very much like the little book—the author's name always escapes me—entitled something like *Everything I Needed to Know I Learned in Kindergarten.*

This author writes the same thing: all that is truly important, what shapes us as humans, is learned in kindergarten. When I've thought back on my little school, it has dawned on me that it was the finest grade school anyone could ever want. The teachers, among whom there was only one male, were for the most part the finest examples of grade school teachers anywhere.

The school is, as it was back then, an autistic's dream. It was the proverbial one-room, red brick schoolhouse. It is a rather uncomplicated shoebox of a building, like my house. It is perfectly symmetrical and neat as a pin. On the first of its two floors were the offices, the library and rooms for grades K-3. The second floor housed the teacher's lounge and rooms for grades 4-6. Off to the side, between the floors, was the back playground entrance/exit and the gym. The smell of the place is what has always stuck with me: I now recognize it as the smell of a clean, new school. The last time I ventured into my old grade school it still had that smell.

I remember the clean little restrooms and the three foot high pegs along the walls where we could hang our coats, and underneath we could leave our galoshes. It always seemed to me, even then, that a wizard or magician must have designed and built that place. Even the bricks looked magical, and set into the side of the then-new school building, next to the main entrance, was the old cement sign which had been part of the old school. It is dated circa 1913, I think, though the school itself was first established well before 1913.

There were odd little rooms and offices, which seemed like conference rooms. I remember the kitchen next to the gym (which sometimes doubled as lunchroom) because I regularly visited with my first special ed teacher in one of them. In another, I was taught how to read and write music by a fine gentleman, who also instructed me in playing the flute. He routinely visited around the grade schools as well as holding a teaching post, conducting the gifted junior and senior high orchestras. I will never forget him, his gentleness, sophistication and intelligence. He always smelled the way I thought a man should smell: pleasantly of soap, a hint of cologne, and the slightest air of tobacco.

He dressed very well, the way I thought a man should dress, and remember, he was the only other male teacher I ever saw up til then. My sixth grade teacher, on the other hand, was an eccentric man with an explosive temper who had seen war (WWII, but we were forbidden by the other teachers to ever bring it up). He was also the first person I was close to, outside my family, who suffered from Tourette's Disease. He and I got along well, and he liked my zest for learning things on my own.

The other students lived in mortal fear of his temper, because he was known to throw erasers and chalk at stupid pupils. A big rumor was that back in the 1950s he had locked one boy in the room's closet; the other big rumor was that he had placed a boy in a large plastic trash can, sealed it, and then kicked the kid down the steps, can and all! I never believed any of it, and never saw Mr. Carlson do anything more than occasionally rail at the students.

All of the teachers were a bit eccentric, and very good at their work. They made the first lasting impacts on me, and as I have mentioned, they instinctively knew how to handle me without the benefit of professional guidance on how to handle a little autistic, ticcing genius. Among these teachers were the "Hispanic Corps" as I call them, the teachers who helped the recently arrived Mexican immigrant students as well as students like myself, those who were more fluent in Spanish than in English. The Hispanic Corps taught me to be instantly fluent in both languages, and no doubt spurred my passion for learning other languages.

We Hispanic students would go into another special room on the first floor, across from the library, a sort of conference room set up like a classroom. It was there we perfected our English and our Spanish. The whole program was amazing for its time: English as a Second Language classes, of course. But who would think of setting it up so the kids could perfect their Spanish as well? That's an example of the school's progressive and capable atmosphere. Many of the Hispanic teachers were on the regular staff—a few of them seemed to be travelers—and I recall them all with great fondness.

All the children at my school were from the same neighborhood. It was like a great family, and I made my only life-long friends at that school. The nature of our gradeschool years reminds me of the chasanim, the little traditional Jewish grade schools where kids learn Jewish history, Hebrew, Torah and Talmud for the first time. It seemed that wonders would never cease when I was in my classes, and, though there were rough periods, I loathed leaving when the time came to leave for junior high.

The only thing I would never miss was the third grade teacher I mentioned. She took an immediate dislike to me, which blossomed into an overpowering hatred. Needless to say, that woman did not last as a teacher very long. Not forgetting her evil character, I researched all the area schools a few years ago. To my relief, there was never again found any trace of her.

Yes, it seems like an idealized picture, but it is not. I have revisited the school many times, tried to keep track of the teachers (most are dead now), and reminisced with friends who went there with me. No, it's all true, and it was marvelous. When I started, my mother or one of my sisters would walk me to school, though I walked back home by myself—the school is three blocks from my house. We had good lunches provided for us, we had the most spectacular fun on holidays, especially Halloween and Christmas.

No wonder my mother always raved about her gradeschool activities, even when she was in her early eighties. She never forgot, and neither will I. Once, and only once, my mother told me about a grade school adventure she went on, I think with her 4th grade class. They went on a breakfast picnic, apparently to a giant park or near the lake. They brought all their little furniture with them (these were still Victorian times in Mexico). My mother enthusiastically told me how they had concluded their picnic by making baskets to take home with them, and later being given hot chocolate and other treats. She had the same warm feelings about her gradeschool years as I had about mine.

Junior and senior high years, for reasons I am not fully capable of understanding, are recalled with much fondness, even tears, by many. Those were among the most miserable years of my life. My only fond memories, other than a handful of wonderful teachers, are of the times I spent alone in the libraries, studying, listening to music and drawing. Of course I had a few acquaintances and a reputation of sorts, but those were negligible consolations.

A reputation is essentially a figment of the imagination, and my few friends are mostly gone, several dead and the rest not in touch anymore. The schools themselves were nothing like my beloved grade school. For the first year of junior high I actually wanted to go back a year. It was like throwing a small-town provincial into Oxford. Not Oxford's quality, mind you, but sheer size and intimidation is what I mean by Oxford—and none of the class.

I want to avoid bitterness in my life and always have, but when it comes to high school (and doctors), I can't help indulging in it. I've never seen a bigger bunch of idiots in administration even in the civil services, and they were proud of it. They even withheld my high school diploma temporarily for skipping a few crummy gym classes. One of those super-ironic twists of which my life is composed, the gym teachers were among the most decent human beings I knew.

The strangest thing of all in high school was that there were many students suffering from various mental illnesses or disabilities, and we all graduated in a collective temper because of the rotten dealings we had with the school—several of us published signed letters of protest. I can only hope that things are better now. Judging from what some parents have told me, they are not better.

One thing I will never forgive is the fact that the assistant administrators at the school suffered from panic disorder. She should have known the ropes, should have commiserated with troubled students, but it was quite the contrary. That woman (if the old battle axe is still living, which I doubt) was one of the meanest, coldest people I've ever had the disgust of knowing. Once she even mocked me to my face in the presence of my parents, and when I had to see her she barely hid her contemptuous lack of interest. Otherwise I really can't blame the schools for not having known what to do with me. After all, there weren't any gifted programs or special needs arrangements. I was really lucky to get the two specialists in grade school, and fantastically lucky to have the therapist.

As a young adult I often ran into some of my old grade school teachers, who practically apologized for what they considered a rather lackluster school environment. That they had held on to such an attitude for so many years is amazing and puzzling—but I can and do blame the high school teachers for their neglect of troubled students. In looking back, it is a source of amazement that no one from our graduating class returned to riddle the building with bullets.

Come to think of it, a boy who was in high school with me was recently arrested for violently raping and murdering a woman. He was a withdrawn, clumsy boy who showed some emotional and learning disorders. It struck me that the poor murdered woman would still be alive if our high schools had been of better quality.

It would be excellent if the high schools had an office of special needs (or Education Services as it is called at the colleges). Perhaps many already do; I don't want to do those schools a disservice. Ideally, the students would be shown respect, they could have an advocate in their fight against disability, and could arrange for special services as needed. More of a pool of ombudsmen, I should think, rather than just an impersonal office staffed with hostile idiots.

Perhaps schools have this now in some dreamland, but judging from the stories I've heard from various parents, it never will be, and wishing will not make it so. It is incomprehensible that teens with problems should be so deprived. I see a metaphor here: parents sending their child to learn the piano, and then finding the worst, meanest instructor with a heap of junk for an instrument.

The taunting finally ended for me in high school, which was another sigh of relief in my life. When I was in school, the eccentric, the rude, the defiant, the nerds and the art-set were the rulers. Prom-queens and jocks only served as wallpaper—perhaps that is justice of some kind. Some might find it hard to believe, but the wide world of sports was not the religion of our high school. In spite of a darned good football team, respect among students was usually paid where due.

Among the student body itself, the artists, thespians, musicians, even the projector operators all had places, and our places were high. As an intellectual, an eccentric artist and musician, I fit into this sphere very nicely. My acquaintances were not too troubled by my strangeness; in fact they liked me for it. If I happened to make gestures, faces, stick out my tongue or give the finger to the teacher, so much the better! How were they to know it was involuntary and sometimes unconscious?

Thus, I learned my first lessons in confidence and self-acceptance. It is natural for almost any teen to find some friends or a social group; but most of the disabled kids in school get nothing. This is what makes me emotional when I remember the last years of high school: no matter who you were or what you suffered, you could rely on friends.

I can remember the time my friends began shouting at a group of teachers on my behalf, because they thought the situation was unfair. There is a vital lesson in this for today's society and for the medical community, as we shall see.

A Professional Nightmare: *Our Medical Community*

Treat your patient's pain as if it were your own.
- Traditional Chinese medical lesson

A great deal of intelligence can be invested in ignorance.
-Saul Bellows

In order to start on the right foot, this seems like a good place to relate the story about how my diagnosis finally came about. It is probably a much more common type of scenario than I think, but it's a valuable story worth telling in full. At some point in the early 1990's I decided that the "war with myself" could be won simply: all I needed to do was to finally, fully accept myself. The psychiatrists I saw off and on for over a decade had been deplorable in their ignorance. All of them had misdiagnosed me, had been completely lost, and were useless to me, with the exception of one. I was through with them.

I determined that I would not just accept but celebrate whatever might be wrong with me. No more medications! This whole new outlook was and still is a matter of survival. I had, after all, invented a favorite saying about myself: "I am at war and it's a fight to the death." Well, I was pretty sick and tired of that saying. This was complete surrender: no more war, no more psychiatrists and no more pills.

Then a few strange things took place later. In our local paper of 3 January, 1992, I spotted an article on Mozart, my favorite composer. Right away I clipped it after only briefly skimming through it, since I file any article of interest in my morgue file—and articles about Mozart are rare. This particular article dealt with the recently proposed theory that Mozart may have suffered from Tourette's Disease. It has always been a source of pride on my part that I know a great deal about Mozart.

Now here was an article, all new territory since I was totally ignorant of TS. In grade school I had discovered that Mozart and I had a number of personality traits in common; it was almost unbelievable to read that those traits happen to be symptoms. We have a brilliant endocrinologist, Dr. Bernard Simkin, to thank for the information. He's the one who first thought Mozart might have had TS, and wrote a landmark paper on Mozart's tourettic and scatological symptoms. His paper had inspired the newspaper article I read.

It would be good to digress momentarily to explain Dr. Simkin's examination of Mozart's symptoms. Dr. Simkin is also a big fan of Mozart's, and he is a cellist in the Los Angeles Philharmonic Orchestra. When Peter Schaeffer wrote his play *Amadeus* in 1986, he had thoroughly researched Mozart's personality as revealed in Mozart's letters along with the letters and descriptions of his contemporaries. So Schaeffer created a theatrical Mozart who seemed very true to life.

Dr. Simkin had been fascinated by Mozart's coprographia (the writing of obscenities and risqué material), and also thought he detected a tourettic pattern in Mozart's advanced and repetitive musical ideas. When *Amadeus* was made into a film, Dr. Simkin, who had seen it, was not yet fully involved in his research. After he began his research, he remembered the film and watched it a second time. It was then that it struck Dr. Simkin that Mozart had to have suffered from TS.

A big deal was made about this in the media. Many doctors scoffed at Simkin, while others confirmed his retrodiagnosis. When Peter Schaeffer was interviewed about the TS diagnosis, he said, "This is the first time I've heard the word 'Tourette's.'" Other doctors were more generous, agreeing that Mozart may have had TS but cautioning against attempting to diagnose any historical figure.

After Simkin published the paper on Mozart's so-called "scatological" tendencies, he published another paper on the feasibility of a Tourette diagnosis—then others followed suit. Soon afterward, the literature on TS began listing Mozart as a famous figure who suffered TS, along with the other historically famous sufferer, Dr. Samuel Johnson.

It was just after clipping the article on Mozart that I read a bit about TS, but I didn't manage to achieve an understanding of it. It wouldn't sink in.

After pondering a few days, wondering if this could be "IT," I wrote in my diary: "I know I definitely do NOT have Tourette Syndrome!" Even at this point in time TS was not and had never been a subject of interest to me. My only interest lay in the fact that doctors were saying Mozart had it. Besides, I knew of no definite resource to study.

What was out there was so thin that I don't even remember what I read; and bear in mind that there was as yet no such thing as the internet. Pending further research, I folded up the article on Mozart and stuffed it in a book of his letters I was reading, the very letters that Simkin had scrutinized. It was a book, it was about and mostly written by Mozart, so I happened to own it. And I loved reading all those silly, tourettic letters of his, which reminded me of my own private writing style.

It was past the middle of 1993 before I made any further pursuit of the subject. To this day I don't know what made me remember that article stuffed in the book of Mozart's letters, and wasn't too sure it was still there. I think what happened was I went to search for the article after seeing some new material on TS, and remembered the book which had been long shelved. When I found it, I opened it and the article fluttered out.

I re-read the article and then the book, noting Mozart's odd writing style and likening it even more to my own. I had read the play *Amadeus* when it was first published, and I now read it again, taking careful note of the tourettic features of Mozart's character. The film version, coming out a few years later, I watched and watched. Suddenly it was from a different perspective: it was like seeing myself, and it was not all that pleasant a sensation. So, after re-reading the article much more carefully, I decided to go to work in earnest.

With a comprehensive list of symptoms in hand, compiled from the Mozart article, the play and film, and some basic TS information, I researched every available piece of information at all the libraries. I also solicited and received a huge packet of literature from the Tourette Syndrome Association; all these materials, which I still have, were the beginning of my TS file. Thinking back on my childhood, I then compiled a list of what I was sure were symptoms. I did a complete medical history of myself, cross-referencing with the list of symptoms I had gathered from the TS literature.

Months were spent remembering as much as possible; I took complete stock of my life up to that point. I pestered my entire family with endless questions without telling them why I was asking, but then they were used to this sort of thing from me. It was also a privilege to talk on the phone many times with the lovely lady who at the time was head of the Illinois chapter of the Tourette Syndrome Association, Lily Frantzell. Sadly, Lily is no longer with us.

The whole process of inspiration, research, thinking and writing was so monumental. I and no one else had discovered what was wrong, just like a scientist or a codebreaker. This in spite of the school system being very uncooperative with me. When I went to the administration building to request all my files, they gave me two lousy sheets of paper. They claimed that all records dating back that far had been destroyed. But it was finally over! All that suffering. All that misery. All those blind alleys. Einstein could afford to shrug and laugh if his research went kerflooey; but in this case the stakes were astronomical: this was my life. I had found the solution: TOURETTE'S DISEASE. It was like finding and deciphering the Rosetta stone.

Then I sought out a doctor, which required months of plain old legwork. At that time I wasn't seeing a physician, so I could get no referral.

What happened when I did finally find a doctor will shock you.

It was early spring, 1994. As I sat on an examination table, I thought the brilliant neurosurgeon, with whom I had a previous acquaintance, was acting a bit too suspicious of me. I explained that I was certain it was TS that had been plaguing me all my life, and hoped he would confirm or deny this without doubt. He had in his hand my type-written symptomological history, that written record of the months of painstaking research, digging, reading, and painful reminiscing.

The brilliant doctor badgered me with some of the nastiest and dumbest questions I'd ever heard. "Why do you think you might have Tourette's? Just because you read about it?" He then proceeded to patronize me even more. He spoke to me as though I were stupid, and yet he sat some distance from me squirming in a chair, as though I might be dangerous. Naturally I became irritated. Here was the great neurologist and neurosurgeon, allegedly one of the best. He had saved a friend's life a few years back, which was how I met him. And now here he was giving me the business.

Judging by the tone of his questions it was eventually quite clear that he knew TS was the problem, yet he wouldn't say it. He kept asking me what I wanted of him, what I expected him to do. He knew the answer! Hadn't I told him? I wanted a confirmed formal diagnosis of Tourette Syndrome, or confirmed formal assurance that it wasn't TS, that was all. It was up to him, and he basically toyed with me. He tried to make me feel guilty for wasting his time and he never, EVER confirmed or denied the diagnosis to my face.

Once we left the examining room, the brilliant doctor made a brilliant production out of writing "ANXIETY" on the diagnosis sheet in big letters; he then tapped the word obnoxiously with his pen, holding the sheet under my nose. "That's your problem. You need to get it treated."

Exasperated, I asked him point blank if he thought I had Tourette Syndrome or not. "Well," he sneered, "you would know better than I would." He added, "You're pretty sure you have the answer anyway." The brilliant doctor had tried to make me feel two inches tall, and made no attempt to hide his unprofessional contempt for me. He actually had the nerve to tell me he was thoroughly "burned out" on his job when I confronted him one last time; as if his burn-out had anything to do with me.

It is all still a mystery to me, but from what I've read in the last few years, this is not an uncommon scene in doctor's offices, right down to the doctor's burn-out complaint. I was so angry with him that I ticced, cursed and trembled for two hours after the appointment. I also immediately made notes about what had transpired, once I had returned to my car, which I later copied into my journal. Those notes comprise the basis of what you have just read.

The weird upshot is that the brilliant neuro referred me to a psychiatrist (remember the complete dolt I mentioned, the one who wanted me to be depressed?). He sent her a letter in which he did confirm a diagnosis of TS. At the end of my initial intake visit with this psychiatrist, she concurred with the diagnosis of Tourette Syndrome, telling me that it had already been made by the brilliant neuro in his letter of referral. To her credit, she seemed little amused by the game that he had played with me.

She never did tell me if she knew something else about it or ever discovered the machinations of it. I've always entertained a fantasy that she must have at least written to the neuro in order to find out why he had behaved so badly. In any event the brilliant neuro subsequently sent me a cold letter informing me that he was no longer available to be my neurologist. Could it have been something I said?

It was at this point I realized that there exists an equation, applicable to doctors, teachers, other professionals and those whom they serve. The equation includes parents as well. It is that in dealing with a patient, there are only two categories of people: the Culpable and the Brave. Sounds trite, but think about it.

After the visit to the shrink, I was positively exhilarated. The curse finally had a name, and thus it had been lifted! After all the galactically stupid psychiatrists blundering around, alternately drugging me or refusing any kind of treatment, this pain finally had a name. The monster had a face! Ah, I had struck the wrinkled brow of the white whale at last! I have to add that since the shrink visit, I've had no less than three concurrences on the TS diagnosis, along with diagnoses of ADHD, dyslexia, Executive Disorder, OCD, and the most recent diagnosis, Asperger's autism.

When I later asked my therapist about the trouble with the neuro, he replied, "Well, you've been misdiagnosed for years. They were incompetent, and no doctor wants to come along later on and label the others incompetent by diagnosing you correctly."

My reply was, "Well, that's not my problem and it shouldn't have to be, but it is. The fault rests with them. What could prevent this from happening in the future?"

"Increase in knowledge...I hope," was the sad response.

This therapist, whom I had been seeing forever until I had to stop, is another godsend. The dopey shrink had asked me if I wanted a therapist and I said yes. My few requests were granted as far as the type of therapist I wanted, and presto!—there he was. He has done me alot more good than all the doctors put together. Bravo for him I say: I had finally found someone that was as brave as I imagined myself to be!

What's Going On Here?: *Diagnosis Problems*

You can't shake suckers out of your sleeve.
-Groucho Marx

I'd like to include a few words about Tourette diagnosis and its problems. There is a definite, minimum criteria that has been established for a tentative diagnosis of Tourette Syndrome. The trouble is that doctors do not always agree on the criteria. A few years ago, doctors could not agree on the number of diagnosed cases because they each called the shots differently. What was Tourette Syndrome to one doctor was nerves or nothing at all to another. The main source of this difficulty has been the disagreement on just which symptoms fully constitute TS and which do not.

Too many mistakes due to all sorts of reasons are made in this arena, and TS has been misdiagnosed all too frequently. Naturally the bulk of the literature is in disagreement, ignoring new findings, with the various experts sometimes actually arguing in print. It's almost like some sort of demented nineteenth century political muckraking. Even the DSM-IV entry is totally revised. Now, the excellent Merck Manual has a good Tourette's Disease entry in its neurological diseases chapter, right between the various choreas and Parkinson's Disease—where it belongs.

The usual criteria goes roughly something like this: onset of tics between the ages of seven and eighteen (when I first began this book the maximum age of tic-onset was 14); presence of at least one motor and one vocal tic (not necessarily concurrent) for at least one year; rule-out of any other possible cause. You won't be shocked to know that even this skeletal criteria is argued.

Doctors have argued the age of tic-onset; they argue about the expression and types of tics; they argue about what Dr. Tourette wrote. One book even got Dr. Itard's first name wrong—in this book he was given Dr. Charcot's first name! Of course this particular book to which I refer was, in my opinion, practically a fraud; the veil of charity shall be drawn over it now.

Another item of interest I want to include is the apparent difference between male and female TS sufferers. It was thought that TS was three times more common in men than in women, the exact statistic seen in high function autism. Now, legend has it that women manifest TS in a different way than do men. Men, the gossip says, tend to show TS more outwardly: tics, violence, odd behavior. Women allegedly "show" less, being more prone to the internal symptoms like obsessive compulsivity and internal tics. Undoubtedly the center of this Gordian knot will show that it is simply a matter of how the individual deals with TS: a sum total of the constituents of the patient's personality.

It has been shown that cultures manifest Tourette Syndrome in slightly different ways, and this reminds us of the difference between males and females. Among many cultures there is more pressure to control symptoms than the average Westerner could imagine. In other cultures the opposite is true. Likewise, men and women would logically have not only different personalities and symptoms, but also complexly different coping methods and necessary ways to deal with those symptoms.

My own symptoms tend to lean more toward the "feminine camp" sometimes, and in light of the research, the doctors are mystified by this. They are mystified for naught; as Dr. Sacks has written, there are as many manifestations of TS as there are people with TS.

One of the hopes I have for this book is that it will integrate once and for all the complete spectrum of TS-autism-OCD. I believe it's easy for anyone to spot even a clinically recalcitrant case of Tourette Syndrome, if they know enough about it. Though I can say I know quite a bit, having researched and studied a great deal, I hope it is very clear that I am not a Western medical doctor.

As a practitioner of traditional Oriental medicine, I have diagnosed many cases of TS over the years, and I have never been mistaken. Still, the first thing I do is urge the person in question to see a competent neurologist. I will not urge anyone to see a psychiatrist, because that is begging for trouble and heartbreak.

All that we really need is to open people's eyes to all that happens with

Tourette's. Then the diagnostic troubles will vanish.

The way things are now, I tremble to think what is in store for a sufferer who goes in search of treatment. Want to know exactly why?

The Doctor Who Was A Monster

Quite some time after the ordeals of my initial diagnosis and follow-ups, I visited another neurologist. Unbeknownst to me, he had a local history of malpractice, but there he is, still practicing to this day. This is the doctor whom the Epilepsy Foundation had sent me to see a decade earlier, when it was thought I had psychomotor epilepsy. Obviously he was incompetent to spot the TS back then, because he was tentatively sure I had epilepsy. Back then he had ordered a full range of tests. They proved I had no detectable epilepsy of any kind.

Later I discovered that this doctor had accused me of ignoring his orders and never having any of the tests done. This time around he had basically tricked me into coming to his office under the auspices of an evaluation: he was heading a movement disorder clinic, and I was informed I would need to see him for evaluation prior to joining the clinic. As it turned out, his plans for the movement disorder clinic blew up.in his face, with only himself to blame.

This guy is a real loser. When I saw him, it was like seeing the other brilliant neuro all over again; and after making the appointment at his behest, he even pretended not to recognize me at all or know why I was there. When it was all over, as I stood at the reception area for some information before leaving, I heard the idiot talking to a nurse. He proclaimed, "That Antonio Hernandez is NUTS!" As I froze on the spot, I overheard what I thought was the nurse shushing him, followed by a sort of pregnant silence.

I could visualize the nurse pointing toward the reception area where I was still waiting, and motioning to the doctor to shut his fat mouth. Then it seemed that there was a sound of sheepish feet shuffling away on the carpet. This is the doctor who later accused me of faking my tics, based on his lively imagination more than on diagnostic acumen. If my two diagnostic horror stories have given you the willies, I'm pleased. These kinds of doctors should give everyone the willies.

A funny sort of post-script to this: Dr. Sacks has written that many TS sufferers either diagnose themselves, or are diagnosed by family or friends;

they then seek a competent doctor for confirmation. But he also mentions that there are quite a few cases in which doctors have been diagnosed with TS by their own patients! I think this is funny, but it isn't really a humorous situation. It adds disheartening support to what we know about the medical community.

I'll tell you this: don't let anyone downplay Tourette's Disease for any reason. If you have it, a friend has it, a relative—don't try to minimize it. If you consult any professionals who do minimize it or dismiss it out of hand, and there are many, RUN, do not walk, to someone competent who truly cares. Though I may be severely criticized for it, I offer some additional advice: don't pay any charges you receive from a professional if that person's idea of treatment is to insult and patronize you. I've done this once and believe me, the twerp in the labcoat got the message… and none of my money.

When I was in high school, the school-affiliated social workers were actually pretty slick. I was tested, sent to several of these social workers, and someone came up with the diagnosis of "obsessive," somewhere along the line. In fact, the social worker who diagnosed me as obsessive also mentioned my "sexual confusion." He must have robbed Peter to pay Paul. The school tried doing what it could for me, sending me to group sessions for troubled students, which were held in school once a week.

There was a very special person from this period whom I'll never forget: the late Dick Schaefer, the social worker who mediated these high school sessions. He helped me through some rough times, even though he never ventured to diagnose me with anything. He was a very masculine, intelligent yet super-sensitive man.

He had a booming voice that he wisely kept at whisper level and a superior sense of gritty humor that melted into tears whenever he reminisced about Chicago's Irish Channel. I lost contact with him during my freshman year in college, and recently discovered that he has since passed away. He did more for me in my senior year of high school than anyone, up until I met my therapist.

Gotta Get Outta This Place:
Coping Practically (Rather Than Practically Coping) with Everyday Pressures

Some knowledge is like a terminal disease.
-Former U.S. spy who was being blackmailed

We know that Tourette's Disease and autism affect life, and that they in turn are affected by life. Beyond the stranglehold they keep on their victims, they expand outwardly into the sufferer's environment. Just as we have come to be surprised to learn that we are more than the sum of our bodies and our brains, with a subatomic universe holding it all together, we realize that we are more than just individuals; we expand into the universe, illnesses and all.

We also know that we are affected by our environment, and so are autism and Tourette's Disease. At this crucible is born a third state, the combined cycle, of illness affecting and being affected by life. It is this alchemy that presents us with perhaps the most serious problems we face as patients. We must cope with the diseases, with the effects on us and our universe. Then we must cope with the resonating results, trying to keep all our plates spinning while standing on a pole. Talk about your karma running over your dogma.

This balancing act in the Tourette Syndrome sufferer's life brings to mind the old woman Dr. Sacks saw on a New York street in the early seventies. He later concluded that she suffered from "super-Tourette's." She mimicked at lightning speed all who passed by her, then mimicked their reactions to her mimicry. Finally she ducked into an alley, where Dr. Sacks saw her mimic, in one violent wrench lasting ten seconds, everything that had happened up to that point. He wondered at how such suffering would possibly allow a person to keep any kind of identity at all.

What astonished him was the crowd that had gathered about her. Indeed, the crowd is what had initially attracted Dr. Sacks' attention. They had surrounded the old lady, gawking and going through a whole spectrum of reactions. It must have been a living hell for the woman, much more than the disease itself ever could be. Perhaps Dr. Sacks did not realize at the time that all TS patients suffer in this way to some degree.

This is an example of the imbalance of TS and life: the woman with her tics, the crowd surrounding her, reacting with all sorts of negativity, compelling her illness to become worse by the second, until she had to run away and hide in an alley. Add to this a puzzled doctor who at the time knew nothing about what was happening. This world should not put the whole weight of such a horror on the shoulders of an old woman—and all of us are that old woman.

In the same vein, I think of all the autistic people who manage to get around, learn quickly, and talk to others. How they are always branded as "nerds" and "geeks"! Even the serious articles that debate whether Bill Gates suffers from autism resort to this name-calling. How many times have you said, or heard someone say, "So-and-So is a clean freak!"? How often do we call people "retards," "clowns," "bums," ad infinitum? These kinds of things must cease. No longer can we plead the ignorance we may have plead back in the 1950s; we cannot even afford to plead the ignorance that the professionals often do.

Long ago there was a television report on a doctor who treats patients with chronic, unexplained back pain and is able to eliminate it. He makes sure there is nothing wrong physically with his patients, then trains them to look into themselves, accept what is happening to them emotionally, and the patients "attack their pain with knowledge." They claim their back pain disappears in a few weeks, all because they regained balance in their lives. It seems to me that it is healthy for TS/autism sufferers, friends and family to take this approach, at least initially.

This physician allows that his patients' back pain is real. He then proves to them that there is no physical cause for it: he thoroughly shows them that nothing is wrong with their physical structures or their health. After this, he gives a seminar on how their bodies are "rebelling" through back pain. Repressed issues, emotions or situations take their toll on the body, coming out in finished form as back pain. He then shows them how to beat it, by simply accepting that the pain is real, the cause is real, but it isn't injury, classical disease or deformity. He shows them that the pain is a physical manifestation of their emotional pain.

Autism and Tourette's Disease would be easy to deal with if a similar approach were used with it: admit that there is a problem, that it is a disease with symptoms and consequences, then move on to deal with it. You would be truly amazed at the people who reject that Tourette's Disease and autism cause problems: doctors of all kinds, educators, employers, families. It is even more amazing how many people would rather just forget the autism in their loved one.

The back doctor reassures his patients first and foremost that they do indeed have a sort of disease, but that it is not what (or how) they thought it was. He tells them that it can be beaten using proper techniques. The same is true of autism and TS... nothing simpler!

Reactions: How We Live Today, Employment, Humor, Friends

It's been my privilege to exist in a society that is not all that bad, contrary to the unpleasant observations and comments I've made thus far; I truly feel that this is the greatest nation ever to exist on the planet. Nevertheless, I do have to tell you that we TS/autism sufferers never fail to panic in some way when we're in public, as someone may well holler at us, poke fun, or react in some adverse way. "Anxiety attacks," did someone say?

Anyone would fear and loathe being mocked, given the bum's rush by store security, having the police called, being whacked by the canes of little old ladies—all of which have happened to me, and to many others no doubt. I'll grant that the worst thing that usually happens is that kids make faces at me, imitate me, or somebody pokes some kind of fun. Believe it or not, I sometimes find these reactions truly hilarious. Though at such times it also crosses my mind that maybe the stupid kid who's doing such a good impression of me has some kind of disability himself.

Reprimands and ostracization are also far too common. Then there are those who regard Tourette symptoms as fake, who think TS belongs in a book about yetis and UFOs, that the symptoms are some kind of ploy for attention. In fact, the need to grab others' attention is a tic of the behavioral type, as Drs. Sacks and Comings have often explained. There are many, including experts, who don't believe in very mild forms of autism.

As always, there are totally positive reactions too. I can assure you that many times when my symptoms are quite pronounced in public, the people around me are very patient and understanding to a fault. Generally they are more puzzled than anything else. Naturally there are the odd exceptions, such as with coprolalia: it is an ugly trend that swearing is commonplace today, and the coprolalic TS person, or the autistic mimicking curses, is caught in the middle of it.

Once when I was settling down to watch a movie in the theater, a group of nice little old ladies filed in to take seats in front of me. Suddenly I let loose with the "f" word, which is another frequent tic of mine. One of the ladies turned to me and very apologetically said, "I'm sorry! We'll sit down as quickly as we can." Though I immediately apologized and assured the lady I had not been addressing her or her party, I felt as tiny as a gnat! You see how even in this kind of situation the ladies tried to be very accommodating.

Much more unpleasant are the harsh reprimands I've received all my life about this cursing. Now, there isn't much you can do about it when you don't know why you do it, knowing only that you cannot stop. When the reason is learned, people don't believe it unless you look like one of those phony-baloney desperate cases on talk shows. But then, I simply smile and swear lustily at such pig-headed people. It's the only dignified thing to do, don't you think?

Tourette's Disease can be so very awful because we are robbed of our emotional as well as physical control. The strain of handling symptoms, the emotional tics, and the negative social reactions all combine to leave us in a precarious emotional state. Having been raised in a tradition of strict emotional control, and following a belief system that teaches full conquering of the passions, I've had the unique opportunity to look at this question of emotion. My main conclusion, what I've been driving at for the last few pages, is that it is about as difficult to handle the reactions of society as it is to handle the disease itself. It is no different for the average autistic.

In losing control of the emotions, the sufferer is actually experiencing one or more symptoms. This has to be accepted as a fact. Too many folks are willing to accept that it's nervousness, capriciousness, meanness, bad attitude, and so forth. A Tourette patient is as prone as anyone to weaknesses of character, but these must be differentiated from symptoms. It's not an easy thing for anyone to do, not even for the TS/autism sufferer.

Also, we must be fair and realize that this is a subject still under examination and research. Even Asperger, in his studies of the autistic children, made particular mention of the deliberate "meanness" (his own word) exhibited by the children. With all due respect to Dr. Asperger, I think he was seeing an instance of what I just described in this paragraph.

What really sends a Tourette sufferer over the edge is being accused of something wrong or undesirable. On top of the hurt this disease brings everyday, the sufferer has to be hurt by being told to stop being a jerk, stop being so nervous, stop being so loud, stop acting stupid, stop being so hyper, stop talking so much, stop being so emotional... that's alot of stops, isn't it? This is only the beginning of the Stop List. It isn't confined to TS, it's seen in autism, even in special education schools with deeply autistic kids.

PLEASE, do the Tourette Syndrome and autism patients of the world a favor: remember our disciplined struggle. Think of what we go through, and the kind of life we've had. Think of the ridiculous impossibility that Tourette and autism sufferers are expected or ordered to do everyday: to stop what is unstoppable. Think of us as the Green Berets of mental and social anguish.

People express great surprise when they discover that I have both Tourette Disease and mild autism, because I manage to be pretty calm and normal in public. The other main reason is that they cannot believe that TS and autism could be comorbid; that's an example of how backward our progress has been. Remember, I have to thank my Kabbalah, Buddhist religious practices and martial arts studies for that.

It could be that the autistic symptoms also contribute to my usual calmness. I would think of it as more of a faux calmness—just a façade of sorts. In any case it's better than bouncing around like a marionette. In consolation, through the years I've met many people who know about TS/autism to varying degrees, which delights me. Some folks are very knowledgeable.

I have to pause here to mention that Dr. Sacks has coined the word "Touretter" to describe us, and I have to confess that I am one of the many who strongly dislike this cognomen. The terms "tourettic," "touretticism" and "touretty" have been used extensively by Dr. Sacks. The fact that Dr. Sacks is a brilliant thinker and word-crafter is beyond doubt; when he uses these words he uses them expertly and accurately. I've used them throughout this book precisely because they are so appropriate.

For myself, however, I insist that the words be used strictly as adjectives, especially when there simply is no other adjective to use. Note that I have coined the term autismicities for the same reasons that Dr. Sacks turned "Tourette" into a pliable set of adjectives. I detest the words when they are used to make Tourette sufferers and symptoms sound like some sort of quaint, eccentric bunch with odd habits, or put it across as an alternative lifestyle. I'm surprised we aren't called "Tourette Players"!

I am a martial artist, a priest, a scholar, a musician, a teacher, a prankster and a hearty eater, but I AM NOT A "TOURETTER"! I hope you'll forgive me for using the Sacks terminology in this book when referring to Tourette's Disease and patients. It really is only for the sake of convenience in this case, and you'll note that I've stuck to my guns in terms of how I use those words.

Going on this little tear reminds me of the comment Dr. Sacks made to Lowell Handler. Dr. Sacks told Handler that TS patients are not ill, that they have no disease. Dr. Sacks told Handler that TS sufferers were merely "neurologically different." Now I am not stating that I entirely disagree with Dr. Sacks. It's just that this kind of politically correct medical doublespeak generally sickens me. In Dr. Sacks' case I think he may have been trying to express an idea for a way out of the ignorance surrounding TS. He was probably just trying to make Lowell feel better.

In saying that we are "neurologically different," Dr. Sacks may have been seeking an inroad to let TS into the minds and hearts of the world—admittedly I'm afraid I simply don't know. Dr. Sacks has never clarified his statement for me.

When I read about this in an article about Sacks and Handler, I have to admit I saw red when I got to the part about Tourette's Disease not being a disease but a difference. Similar asinine ideas have been put forth regarding autism, too. Most recently is the watered-down diagnostic version of HFA, which is called PDD-NOS. There are others who would have us believe that autism is some kind of precious gift or blessing. This is nothing but taking the long way round the barn, and makes me really angry. Denial, denial, denial!

I adore knowledgeable people. There are many, many degrees of knowledge concerning TS and autism, and most folks don't really know that much. Once, at what used to be "my" bar, I met a half-toasted girl who claimed to be a nurse; when I told her I had TS, she cried and told me she was sorry. Apparently she thought TS meant something fatal, or maybe she though I said "Down's Syndrome."

I looked at her soggy drink and quickly realized that she wouldn't have been able to tell the difference. I guess I find that everybody, irrespective of their degree of knowledge, wants to learn more (except for that "nurse," whom I left to her martinis and pool-shooting pals). At least they want enough knowledge to be able to recognize or deal with TS and autism when the need arises.

A nice lady here started a TS support group several years ago. It was late 1994, and I was on the verge of founding a group myself. When I asked around, I was given her telephone number. She had already laid the foundations of a group that eventually gained the backing of the Tourette Syndrome Association. We almost had a northwestern Illinois chapter; we have a northeastern one in Skokie, which is the nerve center of the TSA in Illinois.

Sadly, our group fell through, mainly because we never did get a decent number of adults with TS. We had plenty of parents with TS children; a few kids were even diagnosed thanks to our efforts. Apparently, in spite of lively interest and initially high attendance numbers, not too many people were terribly anxious to remain part of the group. I suppose things have to crumble in time, and that's pretty much what happened with our group. It was a tragedy for our area, and it would be tragic to see this crumbling happen all over the world. In my community, there is essentially no HFA or AS group.

I am presented with another excellent opportunity to take a shot at our medical community. When I was on the group's steering committee, my main job was PR and media relations. Now, just take a wild guess which was the only group of people that wouldn't cooperate or help us. Give up? The local doctors!

We had to import professionals from out of town to address the group, and the local medical offices would not put up our flyers; they didn't even really want us calling on them. They were such creeps that years later, when I was looking for a neurologist, some of them recognized my name and then would refuse to take me as a patient. Denial, denial, denial! To this we can add "STONEWALLING."

This brings me to a subject I wish to treat only briefly: employment. I have lost job opportunities and was fired from my previous profession (in law enforcement) because of my symptoms. This is discrimination, pure and simple. Don't think for a second that it's anything else, and don't endure it. Fight! There is no denying that this discrimination, whether in interview, the workplace, or during the application process, is a violation of our Constitutional and human rights.

There is no excuse for it. Now, if there is no diagnosis or knowledge of symptoms, well, that's why I've written this book. If you suspect yourself or anyone else in the family, even a friend, of having Tourette or autism symptoms, then take a copy of this book with you when you go to do something about it. Don't be afraid to show it to your employer if you are a TS or Asperger sufferer. The nonsense about being negatively labeled is the bigot's problem, not the patient's.

I also advise keeping a strong sense of humor. I can't write or say enough about humor. It has saved lives—mine, many times. It has saved my life too many times to count. TS/autism patients, their families, friends, employers, doctors, barbers, piano tuners and mail carriers should always keep their humor in top form.

I recently met a young man who had just discovered that TS is the explanation for his odd symptoms and behavior. What has kept him going all these years is his beautiful sense of humor and the humor of his loved ones. When I met these people, no one was negative, crabby, long-faced or frowning. I have yet to see anything from them but good humor and affection.

On the other side of the coin is a young man I've never met; I've heard about him from a mutual acquaintance. This fellow was referred to me pastorally, but never contacted me. I had no way of contacting him, and I am deeply sorry for this. He suffers tremendously from coprolalia and violent contorting tics. There isn't anything humorous in his life, and I've been told about how he bursts into tears and physical tantrums because of his symptoms. He is not comforted by the fact that he is gay.

He finds himself always having to beg for forgiveness of the few people in his life, as though he were some kind of errant slave boy. There are only two or three people in his life, and they are all long-faced idiots. It strikes me that he represents Quasimodo to them. I would so very much like to reach out to him, but it doesn't look like this will ever happen. He suffers mainly because there is no humor in his life, and very little tolerance exists for him. There you have it: yet another reason I wrote this book.

I'll never forget the bygone years when I was interested in handguns. Some close friends and I were discussing this topic, and they had me rolling on the floor with their impressions of how they thought I would handle a gun, complete with Pancho Villa attitude, tics and swearing. One of them had me crying with laughter as he performed a perfect impression of me, cornering a super bad guy: "ARF! ARF! Stop! Stop in the name of the $@!#$&*?<!%#@# law!! STOP OR I'LL P-P-P-P-PLUG YA!," the whole time twitching and jerking the imaginary gun in his hands. Of course I have handled guns since boyhood, and skillfully, though I do not touch them now for religious reasons.

My symptoms disappeared every time I handled firearms, because I was well taught to respect and care for them at an early age. Anyhow, there truly is no greater medicine than a good laugh and I venture to tell you that, if you don't have humor, consider yourself dead. (That is one characteristic phrase of mine, which as a law enforcement officer I delivered with an icy, menacing calm when I did have to draw my firearm to stop someone: "One move, consider yourself dead.") Manufacture your own humor for yourself if you have to—you need it! Doctor's orders!

Now, the subject of friends deserves a few additional paragraphs. First I would like to point out an interesting observation: people with TS and even autism tend to make friends with each other somehow. Making so many friends who happen to have TS was an intriguing thing to have happen to me, because much has been written about Tourette patients avoiding each other at all costs. You should know that for a TS sufferer nothing has the potential to set off tics like being around other sufferers.

Undoubtedly this explains the reluctance some of them have to getting too close to one another; I've experienced this first-hand a dozen times. However, there seems to be some natural gravitational pull between TS-affected people. It's almost like being at a party and spotting an old friend. As for autistics, it depends on their level of socialization and comfort with others. Many have no real friends, by choice. My grandmother was one of these types.

I cannot speak as well to the topic of high function or Asperger's autism and friendship because I myself am not asocial. Many autistic people are, no matter how well-adjusted and intelligent they may be. What I do know, having studied the writings of asocial autistics, is that they simply can't bear the presence of others for very long.

This was evident in my grandmother and I've experienced this; for me it is not a constant state the way it is for asocials. The best advice I have in such cases is what I always say: listen to the patient, your friend, who knows better than anyone else. Try to accommodate the person; if you're a true friend, it will be the biggest favor you can do for your asocial autistic friend.

In my life, just in the last six years or so, I've developed close relationships with at least a dozen TS sufferers, most of them undiagnosed or "closet" cases. Only two of my acquaintances are diagnosed; I met them in the support group. The others seemed afraid when they found out that I have it. You really can't blame them now that you know what you know, can you? It has been partially my own doing that I don't actually have too many very close friends or a social circle. It is a very sobering fact that most people can't tolerate watching Tourette symptoms for very long, and the autism makes up for the rest.

Lately I just can't tolerate having to raise the issue of TS and autism when I first meet people. However, I do have hundreds of acquaintances and manage rather happily that way. More than enough has come my way in the rejection department, and I no longer have the fortitude to hop on my TS soapbox. So "not getting thick quick," as Roman Catholic seminarians used to say, is a double-edged act of compassion. It would be beautiful if this could change—but even then the autism would get in the way of social progress.

Once I convinced a (former) friend of mine to imitate my tics, since he had expressed a very deep desire to know Tourette symptoms "from the inside." He had often remarked on the stunning speed of some of my tics and gestures; my physical speed and prowess just seemed supernatural to him. He couldn't get over it, so one day he imitated all the tics I had at the time.

I had to train him how to do them, and teach him to develop his speed—a funny scene, when you think about it—and afterward he said in wonder, "God! That is exhausting!" Well, I say he is a former friend because he ultimately couldn't stand my Tourette symptoms, and he probably saw a bit of himself in my autism. He never was one to face reality. He liked manufacturing his own realities.

This friend and his exhaustion got me thinking about injuries from tics, but chiropractors have that area covered. It is ironic that chiropractors, who are considered by many to be quacks, have quite a bit of knowledge about TS. Several chiros with whom I spoke brought up the subject of treating tic-induced injuries, telling me that it had been a specific subject they had studied in class.

Not being one to withhold my opinions, I think chiropractic treatment is nothing but bone-cracking (we can do this ourselves without even thinking about it) and witch-doctoring. This is a smoke signal: what does it tell us about our run-of-the-mill TS specialists, when bone-cracking witchdoctors know more than they?

That said, it should be obvious that making friends is yet another major hurdle for Tourette/autism patients to jump (sometimes more like a flaming hoop). Of course, we all need to have people in our lives who will tell us they love us as we are, and stick with us through thick and thin. Sometimes we have to build ourselves a "family" if we are alone or unsupported. Could anything be more miserable than a disabled person who is rejected even by family? Yet it happens all the time. Even those sufferers with a very supportive family need to gather around themselves some sort of comfortable social support system.

This is most especially true for anyone affected by autism. Autistic people need special care, whether it be in choosing friends, who to trust, or how to make friends. And of course, this isn't a worry at all when it comes to asocial autistics. In spite of what I mentioned about not having too many friends, I do have a comfortable support system of sorts, and I am grateful for it every day.

Also a great comfort to me is knowing that I am capable of comforting and assisting others: several people have called me their priest. The ache felt long ago is now soothed with the knowledge that I am able to give what I rarely received, and that is not an egotistical or condescending view. That is what I call social empowerment. For those who come to me, that is what I call brave.

Cues and Redirection

Let's look at an interesting set of procedures for dealing with Tourette and autism symptoms, that relate directly to the support network—this is something I learned from Tracy Hearle's *Handbook*. It's known as "Cues and Redirection." A cue is one or more warning signs indicating that a Tourette sufferer is about to lose whatever symptom control he or she has, and this can be easily seen in autism once one is used to the idea. One must be prepared to see the cues.

There are several recognized cues, such as increased tic activity or violence of tics, hyperactivity, restlessness, irritability, temper loss, inappropriate emotional display, or a scowling, angry expression. Even uncontrolled giggling can be a cue (this is a prominent symptom in Rett's Syndrome), as can any combination of these or other symptom spikes. The exacerbating symptoms are identical in TS and autism. I've noticed that when upset, agitated and about to lose control, I demonstrate to others an increase in classic autistic symptoms: muteness, rocking, hand-flapping or other self-stimulating activities—things I normally don't do in front of anyone.

When a cue is spotted, the support person/people must offer distraction or comfort in order to quiet things down; this is redirection. It means redirecting the focus of attention to prevent the loss of control that will surely follow. When I am seen scowling, becoming unduly excited or very irritable, or when I begin giggling and screeching like a monkey, my friends and family recognize these as cues. My redirection can usually be as simple as a reminder to lie down and rest, go to a quiet place, or "get control of myself." Actually, my own program of redirection takes many forms: at times my mother would either go completely silent or leave the room suddenly; these actions were all the redirection I needed.

My best friend will suggest an activity or point out an item of interest that she knows I would like. Sometimes she will jump on me and tickle me, but beware: this is not an advisable redirection unless you know it works. Unsolicited physical contact of any kind enrages most TS sufferers, just as in autism. Some like to be held, caressed, spoken to gently or somehow distracted. Others need to be left alone completely or things will get worse.

Many respond to both types of redirection, as I do. As with autism sufferers, deep, steady pressure is preferable to light, annoying, or fluttering touches. Not even Dr. Sacks or Dr. Grandin know why this is, but it is postulated that any stimulus that reinforces solid contact with the environment is therapeutic. This is really what cues are signaling: a loss of touch with one's environment. This loss is particularly dangerous for moderately deep autistics.

Actually, my "support system members" have it easy for one simple reason: I wear glasses. If they are halfway down my nose or if I continuously remove and replace them, it means "Get away from me!" If I'm simply readjusting them over and over or otherwise touching them as I am wont to do, then the other redirections are sufficient; many of my hands-to-face tics involve my glasses. Also I have the tendency to scrub at my forehead with the palm of my right hand, with the fingers pointing up and spread out; that signals deep anger, agitation or disorientation.

I tend to rub my poor forehead raw within minutes, so when I'm seen rubbing or red-headed, everyone knows it's time to do something. When I'm merely angry, I make a sour face which my mother called "the face of one who has few friends." If my best friend sees this face, she'll exclaim, "You're sour!" This is a routine from some cartoon she watches. I'm supposed to reply by making a really exaggerated sour face and exclaiming, "I'm NOT sour!" Needless to say, this cracks me up—whatever really was sour is sour no more.

This is a subject I can't over-emphasize: it's important to remember that we TS/autism sufferers usually respond very angrily to surprises such as being startled or touched from behind unawares, which I think is due to our spatial impairments and tactile sensitivity. If you are the type of smart alec who thinks it would be fun to sneak up on someone with TS/autism, all I can tell you is that you'd better have a great insurance policy and be wearing football gear when you try it.

The few times that this has been done to me have resulted either in injury or a visit to the hospital—and not for me, but for the person who startled me. It isn't that I'm making a threat, it isn't a reassurance that vengeance will be had. It is a SYMPTOM, and everyone should remember this for the sake of safety. Furthermore, I tend to flail my arms when angry or startled, and people just have to learn to get the heck out of my way!

My best friend does a hilarious impression of me when I'm agitated and angry. She dances around, waving her arms wildly like a serial killer on LSD, babbling like the Tasmanian Devil. I get to laughing pretty hard whenever she does this, because she has a startling talent for physical impersonations.

At my house or with friends, though, there is a standing rule of absolute silence when I'm calming down or working on something. I am totally off limits at such times. My tendency is like Einstein's, to drift completely out of this dimension. Quite a bit of this occurs in autism, but I'm not too sure if this is common with TS. It can only be recommended that if your autism/TS-affected pal or loved one establishes a similar rule or boundaries, please be respectful about it.

Also remember that some tend to be oppositional or belligerent. I assure you, this is what I would call an emotional tic. Does anyone really believe we want to be in such a mood? From this proceeds the anger and irritability. As unsavory as this aspect may be, it must be acknowledged. When it gets this bad, I'll go to my room, head for the library or take a riverside walk when it's warm. It is very necessary for me to stay completely away from people at such times; better for them, better for me.

In considering cues and redirection, there seems to be a clear link to the hypersensitivity often seen in TS and autism. Additionally, for unknown reasons there are some folks who respond better to more stimulus, some to less; some only respond to total sensory relief. It's very important to follow the individual's lead in self-control mechanisms. Respecting their rules will help them to help themselves. I believe that this is the first step to truly constructive redirection: show trust if the person seems to be able to redirect herself or himself. Meddling where meddling is unnecessary and unwanted is the major fault in special education today.

Autism requires careful observation and a firm hand, if the autistic person does not have that higher level of self-control. For instance, many autistic children who have self-injuring tendencies tend to strike at others, very forcefully and effectively. This is usually not deliberate, nor is it premeditated—sometimes it is. These types of autistic children simply don't have the normal injury-sensitivity and pain level that others have.

So it is best to deal firmly with such symptoms, to say "No, you don't hit other people," or to find other ways of intervening the incoming punch—but with calmness and understanding. The point here is to do a sort of reverse enlightenment: make the patient see that others do not feel the same as she/he feels. Make them understand what isn't allowed and why. Their senses can and do handle such information very well, if it is well put across.

Senses

My senses, like many autistic people's, are very heightened except for my poor, presbyopic eyes. Taste, touch, smell, vision, hearing, pain: all are super-sensitive though different senses will naturally differ with each person. Perhaps this sensitivity, along with the perceptual disruptions we examined earlier, are exemplary of the recently named "sensory" tics.

We know that autism, for instance, tends to present distortions in tactility, hearing and vision; in Tourette's Disease, there is mild hypersensitivity spread more throughout all the senses. There is in TS a steady parallel with autism in this regard. Tourettic people tend to be more emotionally or intellectually hypersensitive than autistics, but that is only because someone suffering only from TS doesn't have the social and communication problems that an autistic has.

For me there is a good deal of fussing about laundry detergent, perfumes, deodorants, chemicals, textures and so forth. If any of these aggravate my symptoms, I simply declare them an "allergy." I suffer from certain allergies anyway, so I simply don't give it further thought. Declaring any irritant an allergy is, I find, very effective albeit unorthodox protection.

With other sensory problems, I simply avoid them. This gave me enormous trouble in college when I would skip classes because of some unbearable stimulus. It was probably the fluorescent lighting, or perhaps the stuffiness of the rooms. Sometimes adjustments simply cannot be made to certain environmental conditions, and the TS sufferer should be trusted in making these judgment calls. Steady observation will help others determine what aggravates the uncommunicative autistic person. As with tic substitution and routines, the patient's decision should be the last word, and should be respected.

Dr. Grandin made a stunning discovery, which she discusses in her book Thinking In Pictures: her eyes are so incredibly photosensitive that she can actually detect the subtle light-flicker in fluorescent lighting, a rapid cycle of flickers not found in other types of light. Up til then, no one believed that a human could detect these cycles of flickers, but most if not all autistic people can.

All sentient beings possess a sixth sense: pain. All sentient beings possess a seventh sense: time. A "sense" is defined as any of the faculties through which we perceive the world, experience the world and interpret the world. Is there any sense more exquisite than pain? Is there any other sense that penetrates the other senses so deeply? Pain is the sense that warns us of danger more than any of the others. In considering TS/autism, pain is a vital component.

These diseases assault the sense of pain as surely as the other senses are assaulted, sometimes with devastating results. It is sufficient to note that hypersentience and hyposentience are very notable in TS/autism. Self-stimulation is common to those with certain pain senses that have been dulled; but other pain senses are heightened. Stimuli can cause severe pain to all of the senses, as we see in autism. Then we must bear in mind the other pain sense, the psycho-social pain, caused by the symptoms and our society" reactions to them.

The sense of time is also deeply affected by these neurological diseases. It is very difficult to translate the interference that a TS or autism sufferer experiences in the sense of time. One thing that leaps into mind immediately for me is that often, the passage of time seems to be an illusion. It doesn't seem to happen—perhaps because, as I have told many of my friends, experiences that have not been damaged by my lacunal amnesia feel to me as though they just happened.

On the other hand, I have trouble remembering just a few hours into the past, as though the events had occurred decades earlier. This is a purely neurological symptom, but no one has ever explored it in depth. In the senses of pain and time, there seems to be a link with synesthesia.

What research exists regarding the interference of the sense of time is most pronounced in autism studies. There, the scientists and physicians seem to have located a particular disturbance in the sense of time: learning-memory. Normal humans, even the dumbest ones, learn by rote, by repetition, by experience that is repeated. It seems that some deeply autistic people, including the higher-functioning, cannot learn this way.

In my opinion it is purely interference with the sense of time; since it is possible that autism can cause the sensation of floating in a timeless vacuum, any rote or repetitive experience is immediately lost. Then it must be re-done, day after day. Many special education teachers complain about this seeming lack of progress in their autistic students. Naturally—how can they understand the problem?

To a normal human, the passage of time is taken for granted, it is noted, it is sometimes in itself painfully conscious. To an autistic and perhaps for the Tourette sufferer, the passage of time is distorted. I believe this is related to the discovery that babies cannot pick up on things in this way, either, until they have reached a certain age. This memory-learning trouble is present in all babies, simply because their brains are not yet fully developed.

Could it be that underdevelopment or damage of some kind is responsible for the autistic's sense of time distortions? This could then be related to the difficulties we have in dealing with surprise, change, the unexpected, the unexplained.

Needless to say, I have more trouble with changes, new things and environmental alterations than a misanthropic cat. Unusual odors, foreign objects, lights in a different-than-usual place or any environmental rearrangement cause me almost physical pain. Along the same lines, I cannot tolerate strobing or fluorescent lights, and a sudden decrease in light causes me to lose control completely—again Dr. Grandin mentions these characteristics in her book.

There is a certain type of perfume that old ladies around here like to use. I feel like I'm being buried alive whenever I smell it. On the other hand, incense is very calming for me; but if the smoke gets trapped in my room I again lose control of my symptoms. Other TS patients undoubtedly have highly individualized sensory and time-perceiving problems, if any, and Dr. Grandin in her book mentions "perceptual distortions" (which we also examined) that are sometimes mistaken for hallucinations.

Anyway, for starters I think very soft fabrics are good for TS sufferers, and it is known that all autistic people prefer them; Tracy Hearle agrees. I only wear cotton, and only after the stuff's been laundered at least once. It is reminiscent of Einstein's "allergy" to wool. The same was true of Bill Gaines, and Bill wore pajamas under his trousers—the trousers were always wool, and he saw no reason to change this custom!

I think all of us who are autistic are "allergic" to the strangeness and discomfort of wool… and of change. In any case, it's lucky that Einstein's good friend solved the problem by stopping in an army surplus store and buying Einstein his first world-famous sweatshirt. Frank Jacobs, Gaines' biographer and friend, was the one who finally convinced Gaines to buy cotton trousers. When Jacobs first asked why Gaines didn't do this, Gaines seemed to have never imagined the possibility of changing so simple a thing.

This also reminds me of a funny story I read on the internet. This is a hilarious "wilderness story" that a fellow wrote, about his silly brother-in-law and a trip to the mountains. Apparently the brother-in-law was wearing horrible polyester pants, his favorite item of clothing, and puffing away at his customary stogie. After dinner, the hapless guy dropped his cigar between his legs while telling a corny joke.

The upshot is that his pants immediately began to smolder and became fused to his unfortunate rear end, so he spent the evening sitting outside the cabin in the snow, drinking vodka and feeling sorry for himself. Even as I'm laughing violently at this story, I am simultaneously feeling a shiver of polyester-induced horror.

It's the same with new clothing. There isn't anything more disgusting than wearing new clothes off the rack, no sir! I know this because one day I was out wandering about in the only clean clothes I had left. I received an emergency call and I needed some clergy clothes fast. So off to the mall I went to buy the whole wardrobe: black socks, pants, even a belt. By bizarre coincidence I had in my car a new clergy shirt I hadn't unwrapped yet, and after getting that I ran into one of the restrooms to change. None of this would have even been thinkable to me just a few years ago.

While I was dressed in this getup I thought I was going to lose my mind; and this added to the fact that, like Agatha Christie's Inspector Poirot, any piece of lint on my clothes is worse than a bullet wound. What a magnet black is for floating microgarbage! Anyway, I usually have to keep clothes in plain sight for a few days just to get used to them. If all this reminds you of a cat, you're right on the money.

My home environment is the same thing. Everything must be just so, and it must be unchanged. As I mentioned, this is an inviolable rule, and woe to anyone who changes anything. Then the OCD balances this tendency by adding a cleanliness- and neatness-freak aspect.

My shower and kitchen are especial places of scrutiny and shining tidiness—it is clear why so many "eccentrics" of the past, who were either autistic or obsessive, never let anyone into their homes. I just wish someone would tell me why it has to be like this… this feline hell!….

Environs: Survival of the Fittest

Actually researchers did come up with an answer of sorts, though no one is quite sure about its accuracy. It seems that the part of the brain housing our mammalian instincts could be the location of the sensory difficulties and other such differences that we find in TS, OCD and autism. This "mammal layer" of the brain—the subcortex actually—contains the crucible of our senses, our fight-or-flight response mechanism, our territorial instincts, and our survival reactions. This is a quite separate layer form the "lizard layer" that figures so prominently in physical movement and automatic bodily functions.

Remember the "subcortical storm raging" that Dr. Duran mentioned? It appears that these sensitivity symptoms hearken back to simple mammalian survival. I believe these symptoms in particular gave rise to the new classification "Crypto Sensitivity Syndrome." Dr. Grandin discovered in her research on animal behavior that all mammals behave in this hypersensitive way, and are frightened or angered by changes in environment and routine, just like Tourettic and autistic folk.

Dr. Grandin notes that cattle will be startled and suspicious even if a rancher leaves his hat on a fence. They don't recognize such a change in their environment, so it makes them unwilling to enter that environment—it's simple survival instinct. On the other hand, if there is a hat on the fence routinely, they will react with the same mistrust and fear if they see that the hat is not where it should be. Dr. Grandin also mentions the way antelope will actually follow a lioness, watching her every move in case of an attack.

This brings to mind the hypervigilance often encountered in some autistics and most TS/OCD patients: always hunting about, making sure everything is in place and looking "right." All the senses are on red alert at all times, and changes are the very thing that guides animals in survival. In what is a beautiful example of this vigilance, we may notice how kitty usually "goes on patrol" around the house at night, even if it's just a little three-room apartment. So it seems that, in spite of the human being's superior intellectual and creative gifts, TS, OCD and autism can produce a very mammalian survivalist way of thinking, one that has evolved out of most humans.

Noise is an important subject. Loud or constant noise is like poison to me, and here we are!—living in the worst noise pollution ever known to humankind. Repetitive noises are horrid too, and can trigger some real symptom explosions. A woman wrote of her autistic daughter almost having a seizure while the family was driving around downtown. They had gotten stuck in traffic, and were only moving at a few inches' worth of crawl. It was a pleasant spring day and the car windows were open.

They could not understand what was disturbing their daughter; she was acclimatized to city noise and didn't mind the car. Somehow, after finding a parking space they managed to track down the horrible stimulus that was pounding in their daughter's head: a dripping water faucet in an alleyway. This sensitivity harkens back to the theory of vestigial mammalian survival instincts coming to the forefront in TS, autism and OCD.

Music can soothe the savage beast: people with autism and TS tend to like listening to a favorite piece of music over and over. I'm always careful, since the wrong kind of music can be detrimental. Oldies and heavy metal rock generally make me physically sick (but I do like Goth music, Queensryche and Ratt—so sue me). I will not patronize any business that has loud, constant, obnoxious music rattling over the speakers.

Have you ever been around horses and noticed the effect of even a slight but irregular noise? Needless to say, it would be nice to shoot out the PA system at the mall around Christmas; I have to content myself with staying away. I'll bet all this noise is what makes life so hard for everyone, and A LOT more silence would be positively medicinal for us all. This ties in with the redirective measures, as a quiet environment is absolutely *de rigeuer* for Tourette sufferers and autistics alike.

So many people fail to understand this need to get away, to find some good quiet time; this truly amazes me. Everyone needs quiet time—people retreat for meditation, contemplation, or just to "veg out" awhile. In Judaism, retreat and rest is the main point of the Sabbath, it is one of the ways to consecrate and "make holy" a certain period of time. The same goes for Buddhism.

When it comes down to an absolute necessity, people can be very misunderstanding of our needs, especially in the schools. Since I mentioned Judaism, it is interesting to note that, no so long ago, the Jews were marked as a lazy people because they had that one day of rest, from sundown until the following sundown, while everyone else had to work every day.

Buddhists, too, were considered lazy parasites because they did not till the land. The point is that the Tourettic or autistic person needs a rest from the usual environs, and it is this need that others find so hard to understand. It boggles the mind how people cannot understand something that they themselves need as much as anyone.

I suppose it is on account of the exhausting nature of autism and TS, not to mention most environments, that the TS/autism sufferer needs lots of sleep. As I become more fatigued throughout the day, the symptoms get pretty bad. I usually have to nap. As my best friend will say to me, "Time to put the baby down!" At such times I obediently lie down, and immediately fall asleep. This is nice since I have awful symptom flare-ups at bedtime; I've read that this is very common.

It's probably due to the sudden cessation of light and noise which we have to battle all day, every day. So I have a comforting set of routine rituals to be performed before bed, and these assist me in making the adjustment to the fact that it's bedtime. Again, we see parallels in the animal world. This helps so much that I recommend it to everybody, TS/autism or no!

As I've said, if pain is our "sixth" sense, dulled and distorted by autism, then surely time is our "seventh" one, also dulled and distorted. It strikes me that the passage of time is a problem worth investigating a little further relative to autism. It brings to mind something that Temple Grandin reported: as a youngster, she placed a comb into a small purse just before leaving to go someplace with her mother. She had to keep checking the purse to be certain the comb was still there, and Dr. Grandin noted that the behavior itself took on the nature of a tic.

I have experienced this myself, and most of my touching and checking tics are meant to ensure that something is still where it ought to be. This includes parts of my body, none of which are likely to be moved! Then, the touching or checking naturally turns into a tic. This is thought to stem from a problem with the perception of time flow and succession of events.

It seems that, using Dr. Grandin's example, if she were unable to check for her comb, she could not remain aware for certain that it was there. I experienced this often as a child, and it lead me somehow to think about time travel and teleportation. I suspect it afflicted Einstein as well, and lead him to think of riding on light beams and falling in elevators.

Related to this phenomenon is the symptom I call "freezing." I believe some doctors call it "sticking"—it is the concentrated obsessive attention on a single item. It used to be called "fixation" or "morbid fixation," and naturally these are accurate, if cruel, terms. I have discussed how autistics and TS patients become entranced by spinning objects, such as fans. Freezing is the same principle, and each individual freezes at different times for different reasons.

Sometimes I simply freeze in my tracks, for no reason I can tell. More often I "freeze" on my watch—I mentioned this too—sometimes because the time simply will not register, but mostly because I just freeze my gaze on the watch, and my body follows. I often freeze while speaking, and this is called "blocking." In this case, the freezing is considered a tic.

I'm not sure what "freezing" is, exactly. It leads to tics, and can be caused by tics and obsession. It almost strikes me as a purely neurophysiological symptom, like the Parkinson tremor. I understand that some people who have suffered strokes experience this freezing, and I know Parkinson's patients slowly "freeze," physically. Perhaps there are links between them. It must be related to the time sensory differences we experience, because time passes totally unnoticed and peacefully when I freeze like this.

My best friend happened to hand me a cute little wind-up fan with a lovely holographic rainbow center. Now I am torn between either freezing on this cheap little Japanese-made fan, which is beautiful to me, or finishing this paragraph! Monk and Einstein were often reported as "freezing"; perhaps they were thinking very deeply, as is commonly thought. I believe freezing is a most common symptom, whatever its cause and origin may be. All I know is that it is pleasant, meditative, soothing, and rarely dangerous. I say rarely dangerous—because I had to learn not to freeze while driving!

Naturally the distortion or disabling of our senses of pain and time would be horrifying; but these very symptoms explain the extreme difficulty suffered by deeply autistic people. I believe stress is the first and most powerful effect these causes would have on the autistic person, requiring that every second of life be bound in comforting, recognizable routine—and freezing seems to fit the bill. Many parents of autistic children report that their autistic child will flee even when an unexpected or unusual visitor calls at the home.

On the other hand, all symptoms seem to come to a complete halt when the person is freezing. Intrusions and changes are disruptive to the autistic sense of time flow, scattered or distorted though it might be. Intrusions and changes cause pain in the same way an unbearable noise does. In a way, it seems to be a part of the autistic person's lack of sensitivity, the extremely different than normal reactions, to ordinary stimuli.

Achieving stress and sensory-input reduction is why I have almost always been very spiritually inclined; this is why my routines in daily life are so set-in-stone. You wouldn't believe what a stress-reducing panacea routine can be; and it is top-notch in helping with sensory troubles. Most especially in autism, where even the mildest, highest functioning case can bring horrid distortions of the time and pain senses. This is also the reason I study martial arts. Freezing fits right in there, for there are many moments of natural freezing in everyone's life: stopping to enjoy a sunset, praying, listening to something pleasant, ruminating, or simply kicking back and putting up one's feet.

Of course, routines and freezing can be good for what I call "secretarial deterioration," found commonly in TS: sensory decay/disruption, absentmindedness, disorganization, and trouble handling tasks, some of which are due to autism's hypersensitivity and some due to the various learning disorders.

These problems, on the other hand, are mostly balanced out nicely by my other autistic tendencies, such as obsessive compulsive behavior. Somehow I think freezing assists with such difficulties. Isn't nature nifty?

Synesthesia

Speaking of nature, let me briefly mention synesthesia, which is the "crossing" of senses. In its simplest form, it manifests in some people as the ability to see colors in association with sounds. Tony Attwood has found that synesthesia is very common in Asperger's autism, but I have not seen anything that links it with Tourette Disease.

Dr. Richard Cytowic of Washington, D.C., is a neurologist who has studied synesthesia extensively but makes no mention of either autistic or Tourette patients in his book or his studies. Both Cytowic and Attwood have made a few salient points: they believe synesthesia is an ancient way of perceiving the environment; they believe it provides supersensitivity; and they believe it is possibly a neurological disorder.

My own synesthesia is mild but prominent in my life. My senses all cross, or mesh together. Thus each sense, that is, pain, time, taste, touch, smell, sight and sound, has along with it six additional stimulus-reactions. For every sound I hear, I also experience its flavor, texture, smell and color or light pattern. It is the same with all my senses except vision; I experience no disruption or distortion of my visual field unless I'm very tired. I have had the unpleasant experience of hearing and tasting very harsh light.

So at least in my case, where other people have strictly four senses, I experience at least 16 senses if not more. Then I count the senses of pain and time. In any case, synesthesia is what helped me learn languages and music so well. You can't beat someone who can "smell" or "taste" a wrong note or a grammatical mistake. It also stunted my growth in the more technical aspects of traditional, classical music education. Here again, perhaps freezing serves to "freeze" any unpleasantness.

My cooking is mainly dictated by synesthesia as well—I am an excellent cook. The way my ingredients smell, for instance, has to be accompanied by the correct color, texture, sound and flavor. Once the dish is cooking, I either sniff it or taste it. If the "texture" (that is, the "feel" of it) is wrong, or if it's the wrong "shape," then I have to correct it.

I am reminded of one of Dr. Cytowic's subjects who was a chef. After cooking a chicken dish he sampled it, exclaimed "It has too many points on it!!", referring to the taste; then he proceeded to add some spices. After tasting it again, he proclaimed the flavor "round" enough.

I tend to stick to the same restaurants, and I can immediately sense anything in the regular dishes that has been changed in any way. As an example, I refuse to eat at McDonald's because the food has become very "jagged," very "loud," due to a change in the spices they use on the various sandwiches.

Naturally, people's voices can carry me either into paradise or hell. Some people have voices with incredibly pleasing color, texture, flavor and fragrance. Others are intolerable. For instance I have a friend whose voice, which sounds like that of a quiet newscaster, feels like heavy silk, tastes like burnt caramel, looks somewhat tubular and is plum in color, and smells like rich leather. These are only approximations, since I cannot describe the sensations in any other way.

Newscasters are particularly interesting, if they're good. Their voices generally have qualities like this: the feel of soft cloth, the taste of sweetness, the dark, autumnal, blurry colors, and a deep rich smell. Such voices have an anaesthetic quality to them, and they slow the passage of time. In fact I try to buy my bow ties with colors and patterns that reflect the way I perceive the voices of newscasters.

An even better example is the word "Tourette." When I see it on paper, as with any word, I don't "hear" it in my head the way normal people say they do. Rather, the other senses take over. The same thing occurs when I hear it spoken. "Tourette" is sort of grayish white in color, shaped like a set of asymmetrical but smooth, angular blocks. It smells like soap and tastes like ginger. It also has a nice “movement” or “motion” to it, which some words do not.

This makes me think of what I wrote about talking to myself aloud: I’ve suddenly realized that I think in this complicated, synesthetic way. If I want words or phrases in my thinking, I have to speak them aloud, and that’s exactly what I do, all the time. My reading is usually not bothered, and when I’m engrossed reading seriously, I do not read aloud, though I will often utter certain words I see. In this sense, the utterance is pleasant as well as necessary.

Bear in mind that synesthesia does not entail hallucinations, nor is it comprised of simple literary metaphors as one psychiatrist stupidly suggested to me. Synesthesia is a genuine sensory condition, and some people are actually disabled by it. The other sensory reactions they experience can interfere with the main sensory stimulus, such as the woman who was blinded by jagged red lines whenever her beeper sounded.

I have been blinded while on the phone when the other person accidentally hits a button: the telephone button-tones produce huge green spheres or globs in my field of vision, and makes my mouth taste like dirty brass (remember, I’m a musician, I have actually tasted dirty brass). Synesthesia is a mystical, wonderful gift too, and I generally feel very blessed to be able to enjoy it.

For a clear, complete description of this condition, its gifts and disabilities, read the Russian study *Mind of a Mnemonic* by Dr. A. Luria. This is one of Dr. Sacks’ favorite books, and he references it often. Dr. Luria found a profoundly synesthetic gentleman and undertook a years-long study of him. This fellow, called “S.” in the study but whose name was Solomon, must be one of the most profoundly synesthetic people who ever lived. He was very much like an autistic savant, but did not have too many autistic symptoms.

He had no Tourette symptoms at all. He had a painfully perfect photographic memory, and he never forgot anything. He was tormented by not being able to forget, until he devised a method for mentally “destroying” or “throwing away” what he wanted to forget. His superhuman memory is what attracted Dr. Luria to this fellow, who in many ways was like the Talmudic Innocent.

Solomon was friendly and sociable; he was very anxious to help Dr. Luria understand how his mind worked, and was able to learn more about himself from Dr. Luria’s studies. Sadly, no one knows the true identity of “S.,” in spite of his name being mentioned, nor do we know what became of him. All we know is that he was an attractive, awkward young Russian Jew.

More famous figures who were synesthetes include Andy Warhol, Dylan Thomas, Arthur Rimbaud, Alexandr Scriabin, Vincent Van Gogh, David Hockney, Marc Chagall, Charles Ives, and Piotr-Illych Tchaikovsky. It is certainly no surprise that these famous people were thought to have been autistic, and in some cases possibly epileptic as well.

I have come to find that simplicity in everything, at least as a starting point, is absolutely required. In the next section, we'll explore this idea.

La Vita Semplice: Keeping Life Simple

It may sound almost patently absurd, but it is important to bear one thing in mind: keep life simple, or at least as simple as possible. With all the dizzying facts, anecdotes, horror stories and happy vignettes you've read in this book, it seems that the things we need to learn about TS and autism are endless. But life can go smoothly, really. Dr. Grandin said the same thing in her book on autism; she also mentioned that parents ought to be more confident in themselves when handling the many crises of their disabled children. We can start by fully accepting the Tourette Disease and/or autism in front of us or within us.

I am reminded of a severe symptom I was having that was ruining my life. You know me by now as a big film connoisseur, and when I started having horrible attacks and fits in the theater, I thought life was close to being over. One day my best friend said, "I think your senses are somehow overloading or reacting violently when the house lights go down. Why don't you try closing your eyes beforehand, let them get used to the dark? Then open them after the lights are down."

Her advice was followed religiously, and I have had no trouble since. See how simple? The true secret of its success was that my friend didn't say, "Stop acting like an idiot," or, "What the hell's wrong with you?" She kept her head, accepted the problem, then solved it for me on the spot. I was just too disabled by the symptoms, too agitated to think of a solution for myself, you see.

In the face of what can seem to be a horrible monster like autism, TS or any of the other conditions we've studied, it is extremely difficult to keep one's head. Remember Dr. Grandin's cattle studies? She says that cattle will notice just one tiny little thing out of place or "not right," and they're ready to stampede the hell out of there! It seems the complexities of life and coping will eat us all alive—but it just isn't so.

We stand at the threshold of a new world and we must be brave new citizens, not just frightened cattle. We will learn the ropes because we have to, but we must be willing. The spirit has to be in place for the task. Have you ever seen the problems in a workplace with a person who doesn't want to be there? That person is always agitated, never learns, never fits in, never memorizes the "territory," becomes ill, and certainly never gets ahead. It can get that bad, living with TS, autism and any other disability.

We have to have the courage to dive right into it, or it eats us alive!

"TOURETTE SYNDROME."

"ASPERGER'S AUTISM."

I sincerely hope these have become household terms for you. There are so many, many people in pain, undiagnosed, hiding themselves away because of all sorts of bad experiences. Many are just plain uninterested. This must change, and it is a change for which I desperately hope. Some progress is evident, but not nearly enough. Who can claim even a fraction of the knowledge for AS and TS that exists for cancer and diabetes?

Yet the information is out there, in one form or another. People just don't want to be bothered, and the information is not disseminated correctly. Please, I implore that this little section at the end of the book not be misconstrued as sermonizing (or as my dear friend Chris put it, "It's rather preachy, isn't it?"). A bit of preaching, a bit of sermonizing, perhaps, but very, very necessary.

I've mentioned how Samuel Johnson's friends understood and defended him. You read about how American Natives honored anyone who was different. You read about the Greeks who recognized Tourette's Disease and autism as physical diseases. You will remember the Zulus who look upon TS as a blessing of the gods. Note also that good war-time rules of conduct (note the Geneva Convention) always and everywhere include the strict instruction that disabled people be given deference and preference.

There is also the care and consideration which Doctors Itard, Charcot, de la Tourette and Asperger gave to their patients. Dare we ignore the danger in which Dr. Hans Asperger found himself, studying and caring for patients who were supposed to have been exterminated? Dr. Oliver Sacks has written about the earliest described case of Tourette's Disease (pre-Christian Greece), and there are many more historic instances in which autism has been described. The conditions go back to humanity's beginning.

It would be wonderful if we could gain some more insight into earlier or more exotic attitudes. One fact I did not mention is how some countries pathetically attempt to deny the existence of disease among their own people, such as the Communist Chinese and the Japanese.

Now you know. You also know how Tourette's Disease/autism sufferers are outcasts from their schools, families, societies, and places of employment. You are aware of how Tourette's Disease itself is an almost taboo subject in some medical circles, and how in other circles its existence is categorically denied or ridiculed outright. You know that for centuries in the West, right up to the present, Tourette symptoms have been considered signs of demonic possession.

You are also painfully aware of the tendency to categorize Tourette sufferers as insane or villainous. The labels of "hopeless," "profound," "unreachable," "unteachable" are stuck with a sort of mad glee on autistics. To this day, many autistics are shoved into institutions and forgotten. Remember, my first serious job was in one of these places. It is something that I will never forget.

Now, most significantly of all, you realize how much plain ignorance and even malice there is added to the stupidity and the conspiracies of silent denial. Dr. Sacks' comment that we have a "soulless neurology and a bodiless psychology" addresses beautifully the problem of caring for the individual person. Any developmental disability, any disease, any condition, has behind it a HUMAN BEING. No matter how far gone, no matter how deeply buried, no matter how alien to society.

Such persons are not brain-dead, lying in a hospital waiting to be unplugged. We have actually popularized the failure to recognize the humanity of the disabled: remember the "Elephant Man"? How many people know that his name was John Joseph Merrick, that he was a very sweet, well spoken, friendly and incredibly gifted young man, a poet, engineer, architect and artist, who befriended the royal family and who did not live to see the age of 30?

Even if you did know these facts, what came into your mind when you saw "Elephant Man" either just now in your imagination, or when you saw the play or film? Did you see Joseph Merrick, the lovely young man, or a creature, an "elephant man"? You see: there is a human being there, and you may not have noticed that! What is Joseph Merrick's most oft-quoted remark? He said, I am not an animal! I am a human being! Less known and far more suitable is a verse from a poem he wrote: "The mind is the measure of the man," not the illness, not the disability, not the disfigurement.

We try to turn away whenever we can in the face of disability. No one did Franklin Roosevelt any favors when they overtly and clumsily turned away from the sight of his wheelchair or leg braces. This failure to see the person is a clear indication of barbarity. If, for example, you study the profile of a mass murderer or serial killer, you will see that the most prominent characteristic of such a person is the failure to acknowledge the humanity, the human stature, of his victims. The victims, in other words, are not real people in this kind of criminal's mind.

Therefore, how hard can it be to torture and murder a "subhuman" object? Thus the murderer divorces himself from the crime, from his responsibility, and from any feelings of compassion or connectedness. This criminal will usually de-humanize himself to escape the fact that he is de-humanizing and destroying innocent people. Doesn't it seem that this attitude is creeping into the medical community and society in general? Aren't the disabled always the habitual victims of this parallax view?

Another good illustration of this barbarity is Adolph Hitler's dream of a perfect nation. We all know that the first people he exterminated were the "subhuman, non-contributing" ones: the gay, elderly, disabled, infirm, and poverty-stricken. Hitler is to thank for Dr. Asperger's unpopularity and subsequent plunge into oblivion. After all, wasn't Asperger Viennese, working and researching at the pitch of World War II?

Anyone who had heard of Asperger would have never spoken of him; he might have been thought to be another Joseph Mengele. People might have believed that Asperger was like Hitler: study the disabled, then annihilate them. In Hitler's crazy eyes, the gay, the disabled, the elderly, the handicapped weren't people at all. They were worse than garbage, leeching off society and causing the "normal" people to suffer. Hitler wanted them thrown out like so many Hefty garbage bags.

There was an article some years back in the *Reader's Digest* magazine about how college students in a certain class had refused to condemn Hitler and the Nazis. The article alarmingly referred to the "moral ambivalence" of these students, who refused to pass a hasty judgement on Hitler or the Nazi movement. I ask you, can it be any clearer that we are heading in this repugnant direction as a society? Think about it.

The first step, whatever it is, away from barbarity can carry throughout the universe. Away we would go from the darkness. In the flyers I designed and distributed for our Tourette Syndrome support group, a simple motto blazed across the page: "TOURETTE SYNDROME: LET'S SHED SOME

LIGHT ON IT!"

It is my hope that this book has accomplished that, has shed some light, at the very least. The same holds true for any disease, impairment or disability. Let's shed some light, some understanding, on them!

Afterword

I have a special little afterword-prelude: the lady physician who diagnosed my autism was compassionate, learned and friendly. She erased any doubts about the diagnosis by secretly testing me throughout the office visit, checking to see if I demonstrated the typical autistic lack of response to social cues and body language.

In other words, she was communicating with me intensely but nonverbally, and I as per usual was oblivious, absorbed elsewhere, concentrating on her office, her clothing and voice, the carpet and my fingernails instead. I "passed" her secret tests with flying colors. Thank you, my dear and most out-of-the-ordinary doctor, for seeing what no one else wanted to see, and for having the courage to diagnose it.

I hope this journey, this odyssey, has been as interesting and enlightening for you as it has been for me. I really hope you are now looking through the glass clearly; I hope you've gone beyond the glass. In reading this book, you've basically lived through Tourette's Disease and Asperger's autism (if you haven't already, in some other way). You have even learned a little bit about everything else, thrown in as I went along and learned it myself, for good measure.

Perhaps like me, you've learned many new things along the way on your own. You have the right to be proud and happy about this new knowledge. The estimated two to three million Americans presently affected by Tourette's Disease will certainly feel happy about it, and all those undiagnosed cases will be intrigued by this happiness!

(Don't be confused by the millions figures; they represent a possible total. At present there are only approximately 200,000 diagnosed cases in America.)

That happiness will catch, infecting the one-in-fifty suffering from autism—and hopefully affecting the other 49!

This book really started with a dream I had years before I was diagnosed. It was the most intense dream I can ever recall. In it was my grandmother; she and I were standing by a road near a ravine. We were on our way somewhere, in a countryside that looked like Texas; we stopped to get out of the car and look at the sky.

In the distance we saw ominous black, grey and purple clouds churning horribly, rolling toward us and shooting phosphorescent green lightning. When we looked down into the ravine we saw the clear blue sky with a few white clouds, lying there instead of being where it should have been. I asked my grandmother, "Gramma, are we at the end of the world?," meaning both metaphorically and geographically.

My grandmother, who was a very mystical woman, a devout Catholic who was more like the Jewish tzidduk or saint, turned to look directly at me and replied, "You know where we are." It was as if she was telling me I would soon discover the secret of the awful storm coming, and that I would conquer it. She was quite right.

That storm is Tourette and autism, and I have understood. It has been conquered. Thank you, Grandmother.

Deciphering Symptom Terminology

There are many terms we've covered in this book, despite my promise not to be too technical. (I can be devious that way.) I think it's important to have a guide to consult or simply to skim. There are many terms for symptoms found in both TS and autism yet these have never been simply outlined. The information is certainly out there. You should feel confident that, even though no one really cares much about having all the definitions down pat, you will more easily understand them after reading this book.

I want only to briefly point out a group of prefixes and suffixes which will guide you on the path of tics and other salient symptoms.

The prefix echo- is meant to imply the mimicry of others, whether physical or vocal. The prefix pali- is meant to imply self. The suffix -lalia is meant to imply vocal activity; the suffix -praxia implies physical activity. Thus you see the term echolalia, the vocal mimicry or repetition of others; palilalia, the vocal repetition of self; echopraxia, mimicking others' movements; and the new terms I've coined, dyslalia, meaning verbal dysfunction, echopersonae, meaning the total mimicry of others, and palipraxia, meaning to mimic one's own movements.

With the knowledge of these components, you'll be talking better than the so-called professionals in no time!

Acknowledgements

If it were not for my beloved and oft-mentioned best friend, "Boo," a.k.a. Christine Weber, I'd have been pushing up daisies a long time ago. She sweated right along with me through this whole book-producing process, which took a total of five years to complete.

Bringing me cigarettes, something to eat and drink, helping me in my titanic struggles against symptoms, or just listening to my inane yammering and my reading portions of the manuscript, I couldn't have done a thing without her. This book was written on her computer.

My dear mother, María del Transito Herrera Hernández, may she rest in peace, died on March 3rd, 2000, after a brave and blessedly short battle with cancer. She went too soon, even though she was almost 84, and I never forget her even for a second. She was not only a terrific homemaker; she was a wizard at tailoring, seamstressing, the fussy art of embroidery, and fashion design. She was also a splendid amateur inventor—something else she handed down to me.

My grandmother, my mother's mother, María del Refugio Gamiño Ortiz, passed away on June 3rd, 1985, at the age of almost 98, may she rest in peace, was a great teacher and natural philosopher. She literally and figuratively carried in her veins the best of the Jewish, Catholic and Zen Buddhist traditions. Everyone in our family, including the atheists, considers her to be a saint, and she taught her two daughters, my aunt and my mother, everything they knew. I doubt I would have grown up properly human without her.

My wildly Tourettic aunt, my mother's sister, María del Guadalupe Herrera, passed away on June 27th, 1997, also at the age of 83, may she rest in peace, was the one of the strongest people I ever knew. She was a real friend to me. Without her to show me the way, I would have developed no backbone. Dr. Albert Schweitzer received a student in Africa who wished to study philosophy. Dr. Schweitzer put the boy to work building a new road for Schweitzer's hospital. "If you're going to be a philosopher," Dr. Schweitzer said to him, "you're going to need a strong back. How better to build one...?" My Aunt Guadalupe gave me the strong back I needed.

May all these people who are gone from us be of blessèd memory, and may their memories continue to be for blessings upon us.

A few experts deserve profound thanks for their massive contributions to this work, and to the fields we've studied: Dr. Georges Gilles de la Tourette, Dr. Hans Asperger, Dr. Oliver Sacks, Dr. Temple Grandin, Dr. Tony Attwood, Dr. Lorna Wing, Dr. David Comings, Dr. Uta Frith, and the countless others who teach us new things every day.

Finally, to all the great people who suffer from TS, autism and other disabilities, live with it everyday, research it and lead us away from darkness:

To you I say, as the little alien in an old "Calvin and Hobbes" comic proudly says of himself, "IT WAS I WHO CHOSE THE LANDING SITE. KUDOS FOR NAVIGATOR NEBULAR!"

About This Book's Title

At Wyatt Earp's hearing of 1883, at Tombstone, Arizona—after the famous 1882 streetfight which is known today as the OK Corral Gunfight—Judge Wells Spicer found Wyatt Earp and all pertinent parties to be absolutely guilt-free of any wrongdoing. That Earp and his two brothers, along with John "Doc" Holliday, were dragged before the court in the first place is ludicrous. The Earp brothers were acting law officers on duty, and Holliday had been conscripted at the spur of the moment, if not actually deputized.

The Earps and Holliday were about to disarm illegally armed known criminals, when several of these criminals made the mistake of attempting to draw their guns on the Earp group. The officers of the law had no option but to open fire on the criminals.

Because of the questions of whether the Earps had used undue force, and whether they had committed cold-blooded murder, a hearing (called an "inquest") was held. It was bountifully clear that the outlaws had been openly threatening the Earps for close to two days; these vicious, murdering criminals were stalking the streets fully armed—a crime—on the day of the streetfight.

The Earps, especially Wyatt, had no choice but to conclude that, if nothing else, they had the right to defend themselves on the street. During testimony Wyatt blithely but cautiously pointed out that, in the end, the Earps were better with their guns than the bad guys were. This was a necessary point to make, as the criminals had been basically baiting the Earp brothers.

Judge Spicer, a fine, courageous judge who is underrated in today's world, ruled that the Earp group had "no duty to retreat." That is, under an old English law which had stood for some time in the U.S., a citizen or group of citizens under attack had first and foremost the duty to retreat, in any way possible. Judge Spicer made it clear that the Earps, acting under color of authority and furthermore in self-defense, had no duty to retreat—they had to stand and defend themselves with deadly force.

The concepts of Duty to Retreat and No Duty to Retreat are essentially forgotten today as separate points of law in themselves; each state's laws of self-defense include aspects of both views to some degree. Strangely, just as these law concepts vanished (into the thick rhetoric of statutes), so did Judge Spicer: he apparently wandered into the desert on his way someplace and simply disappeared. He was never seen again.

Afflicted and disabled people, in my view, have NO DUTY TO RETREAT from any of the attacks or challenges they face. Personally, I have gone so far as to make "No Duty to Retreat" my personal life philosophy. So, aside from Captain Ahab, who was not a real person, whenever I face a struggle I often think of Judge Wells Spicer, Wyatt, Virgil and Morgan Earp, and "Doc" Holliday, who were all very real and very brave men.

And I find that there is never any reason for me to feel a duty to retreat.

The Promised Bibliography

As I imagine you've guessed, I have big, fat files on Tourette's Disease, Asperger's autism and autism in general, and also some video tapes and books. There's even a separate file, sort of an "X file" where I keep the weirder stuff, the fringe, controversial, cryptological and just plain nutty. The need for Tourette and autism affected families to keep up with the field should be obvious, and this means literature, literature and more literature (or as with me, a not too shabby though stubbornly quirky memory. Remember, I practice Asimov's philosophy of avoiding false modesty).

This won't be one of those painful bibliographies such as you see in textbooks. I have a personal aversion to such academic platitudes, though you have without doubt noticed that I don't mind using long-winded, useless words and horrid paragraphs in my writing. Therefore, in most instances I have listed only the author and title of the work. I've also followed every entry with my own commentating notes, pertaining to content, availability, origin, and further resources.

The list includes only my favorite materials in no real order, some of which may very well be impossible to find—especially the films and videos. In that case, it is good to remember that a visit to the library—and a phone call or letter to the Tourette Syndrome Association or Autism Society—will net you all the literature you could possibly want. Don't forget the hospitals in your area, which may have excellent libraries.

As I like to remind people (against my better judgment) don't forget the internet. There's a lot of garbage in there, and there is no such thing as the deep web, only deep poop. Still I managed to find great quantities of indispensable information—not to mention some terrific bow tie manufacturers' websites.

To that end, finally, there are no website citations: citing them is a waste of time and one can do better by simply generating a thorough search-engine investigation. I did not even list my favorite bowtie websites; I almost had to be physically restrained from doing so....

About Tourette's Disease

BOOKS:

Advances in Neurology. V. 35, 1982. NOTES: This rather dated (and short-sighted) book is nevertheless one of the most comprehensive histories of the delineation of a disease. It gives a comprehensive, chronological list of the research and resulting publications on tics and Tourette Disease, reaching as far back as the 1820s. Unfortunately, there seem to be quite a few errors, common at the time, with respect to certain symptoms and their proper classification. The other major weakness of this text is that it contradicts de la Tourette himself, in areas which we now know he was quite correct.

Sacks, Oliver. *The Man Who Mistook His Wife for a Hat.* NOTES: Chapters: "Witty Ticcy Ray" and "The Possessed." These chapters stand out as the first modern essays about TS. Though given to a bit of overboard speculation, Sacks paints a vivid portrait of TS, rarely matched by anyone.

---. *An Anthropologist on Mars.* NOTES: This contains the revised and annotated version of Dr. Sacks' article "A Surgeon's Life." Also has the chapter on Dr. Temple Grandin and autism. Dr. Oliver Sacks' extensive article work can be found in the British medical journal "The Lancet."

Hearle, Tracy, Ed. *Children with Tourette's Syndrome: A Parent's Handbook.* NOTES: An indispensable guide packed full of reference materials, suggestions and quotes. This is a Woodbine House Publishing Special Needs Collection book, and the full library is well worth owning.

Shimberg, Elaine. *Living With Tourette Syndrome.* NOTES: Personally, I found this book rather pedestrian and tiresome. I would be so bold as to offer the opinion that Shimberg simply strung together all the popular pieces on TS she could find—and not very well done at that.

Comings, David. *Tourette Syndrome and Human Behavior*. NOTES: Dr. David Comings of the City of Hope Clinic in Duarte, California has been an extremely influential researcher in Tourette Syndrome. Although the citation I've used is my favorite of his books (and the only one I've studied), he's written quite a few works, including an absolutely comprehensive text on symptoms and etiology. His book on tics is an absolute necessity: Comings helped identify several previously unknown tics. A good college library should have his writings; if not, they shouldn't be hard to locate in the "Medical Index" or "Journal of the American Medical Association" (JAMA).

Boswell, James. *The Life of Samuel Johnson*. NOTES: This bibliography may be starting to resemble a literature class list; still, anyone interested in the true exploits of a successful Tourette sufferer cannot pass on the chance to read about the first well-known TS patient in history.

Spitz, Herman H. *Nonconscious Movements: From Mystical Messages to Facilitated Communication (Erlbaum)*. NOTES: This book is in essence a modern study of healthy, normal tic behavior as originally discovered by Chevreul. It is interesting to note that both this book and Chevreul's research were intended as a debunking exposé of "paranormal physical activities."

Robertson, Mary and Simon Baron-Cohen. *Tourette's Syndrome: The Facts*. NOTES: A very nice, shortly written reference book—delivers exactly what the title promises. It is a bit on the simple side, but it should be in any TS library.

Bruun, Ruth and Bertel Bruun. *A Mind of its Own*, Tourette's Syndrome: A Story and a Guide.

Waltz, Mitzi. *Tourette's Syndrome: Finding Answers & Getting Help*. NOTES: This is a terrific reference book, containing dozens of resources in its lists. I like this book because it goes neatly into the research and evidence regarding the link between TS and strep infection. It is also one of the most organized in addressing comorbidity in TS, and makes a strong argument for the link between autism and TS. Finally, this book has one of the finest chapters on illnesses usually found along with TS, including Asperger's autism.

Cytowic, Richard. *The Man Who Tasted Shapes*. NOTES: An interesting, if rather trite and drawn-out, study of synesthesia. It is in fact the only book on synesthesia at present. There is an attempt at diagnosis synesthesia clinically, and a five-point set of characteristics that 'true' synesthesia must have. It has a few short connections with TS, and very interesting perception studies. The very strong points Cytowic makes have to do with very broadly applicable areas of diagnosis; there is an excellent passage, for instance, where Cytowic criticizes doctors for treating headaches, even when there are no symptoms. But something like synesthesia, he continues, they dismiss as 'imaginary'. So there is invaluable general advice Cytowic offers that a lot of neurologists should take to heart.

Von Rilke, Rainier Maria. *The Notebook of Malte Laurids Brigge*. NOTES: Dr. Sacks cites this little tome by the great poet. Though I have not read it, it's worth looking into, to read what Sacks calls "…a vignette of a manneristic ticqueur, …in the streets of Paris. In any case, Rilke is well worth reading no matter what, for in his writings I find a sort of inward-facing, almost autistic wisdom seldom to be found in a poet.

Melville, Herman. *Moby Dick*. (I know—not really very pertinent, but darned good!) NOTES: Anyone interested in the dark side of obsession must read all about Captain Ahab—and take note of his healthy counterpart, the story's narrator, Ishmael.

ARTICLES:

Sacks, Oliver. "A Surgeon's Life." *The New Yorker*, 16 March, 1992. NOTES: Canadian surgeon Dr. Morton Duran, who goes by a pseudonym in the article, is one of the classic examples of a successful Tourette Disease patient. The intense similarities evident between Dr. Duran's TS behaviors and certain autistic behaviors is stunning, though Sacks does not seem to notice.

Phillips, Mark. "Possessed." *New York Times Magazine*, 4 July, 1993.NOTES: A rather phantasmagoric picture of TS in children; Phillips has written about his son, and discovers to his horror that he himself has TS as well, which he notices in the mirror for the first time. An excellent psychological-impact study.

"MOMA When It's Jerking." *New Yorker*, 10 April, 1995. NOTES: A hilarious observation of things gone awry at a Tourette Syndrome conference. A must-read for adult TS patients, especially the side-splitting exchange between "Eric," a well-known conference attendee, and another belligerent TS patient who seems obsessed with bad dogs.

Bliss, Joseph. "Sensory Experiences of Gilles de la Tourette Syndrome." *Archives of General Psychiatry*, December, 1980. Pp. 1343. NOTES: Though this paper is at times torturous reading, Mr. Bliss, a non-professional who took a shoebox full of decades worth of scrap-paper memoirs and turned them into a scientific paper, offers an insider's experiences. It is thorough and detailed, the first work of its kind in the field of Tourette Disease.

Chevreul, Michele. "De la baguette divinatoire, du pendule dit explorateur et des tables tournantes, au point de vue de l'historie, de la critique et de la méthode éxperimentale." (Of the Divining Rod, the Explorer's Pendulum and Turning-Tables, From the Point of View of History, Critique, and the Experimental Method.) French Academy of Sciences, Paris, Mallet-Bachelier, 1854. NOTES: A startling and truly ground-breaking study, which was almost not given to the world and was then completely ignored when it was published. The paper, in expert scientific methodology, explains the urge and tendency to tic that is found in all humans. Further, it explains exactly under which circumstances these tics emerge. This paper is also a must-read for any student of neurology. Bear in mind that the complete English translation of this citation can be found only in the following citation:

Spitz, Herman H. and Yves Marcuard. "Chevreul's Report on the Mysterious Oscillations of the Hand-Held Pendulum: A French Chemist's 1833 Open Letter to Ampère." *Skeptical Inquirer*. V. 25, No. 4, July/August 2001. Pages 35-39. NOTES: This excellent article contains the first complete English translation of Chevreul's original "open letter" essay cited above. It is an absolute must-read, and well worth obtaining by any means necessary. Without this magazine, which my dear Boo picked up for me at an airport, I would never have had access to Chevreul's complete paper.

FILMS/PROGRAMS/VIDEOS:

Twist and Shout. Dir. Laurel Chiten. Narrated by Lowell Handler.

Documentary, 1996. NOTES: This excellent and most recent major documentary on TS is incisive, thorough and deeply disturbing. Chiten has worked hard to present us with the horrifying expanse of super-severe TS symptomology, and it also happens to contain the last interview and film appearance of the late Adam Ward Seligman.

The Tic Code. Dir. Polly Draper. Stars Gregory Hines and Polly Draper. Drama, 1998. NOTES: Polly Draper, whose producer/husband has TS, brings lively and endearing characters to life. She plays the hapless mother of a pre-teen boy with TS, who befriends a jazz musician who also suffers from the disease. The way the musician (Hines) copes with his relationship, with himself and his illness, is also beautifully presented as his character comes to appreciate how the boy's mother and the boy deal with each other.

About Asperger's Autism and Autism in General

BOOKS:

Grandin, Temple. *Thinking In Pictures*. NOTES: Excellent insights and facts dealing with Asperger's Syndrome and HF autism in general. Also presents a fascinating study of livestock handling, Dr. Grandin's field of specialty, and how her autistic thinking made her successful. No one interested in autism should pass on this excellent, concise book.

Powers, Michael D., Ed. *Children with Autism: A Parent's Guide*. NOTES: Another Woodbine House Special Needs Collection book, with a rather anemic foreword by Dr. Temple Grandin. It also includes the first edition foreword by Beverly Sills Greenough. Generally it has excellent though somewhat watered-down data and information. I have noted that the Special Needs Collection, and even Woodbine House itself, tend to be rather uneven in quality (and content) control. This particular book especially seems to waver between the practically inaccurate and the downright simple-minded. With such an important library constantly in print and with excellent circulation, I would think the publishers would be more careful with their materials—but I still think the whole collection is valuable to own.

Ledgin, Norm. *Diagnosing Jefferson: Evidence of a Condition That*

Guided His Beliefs, Behavior, and Personal Associations. NOTES: Not strictly a conventional biography, though by no means a bad one, this book is perhaps the finest existing exposé of autism and its impact on life. It is, however, rather badly and clumsily written, with the wording somewhat difficult to follow and the ideas not too clearly presented. Perhaps this was simply a draining book for Mr. Ledgin to research and write; his son, Fred, suffers from AS.

Trevarthen, Colwyn, Kenneth Aitken, Despina Papoudi and Jacqueline Robarts. *Children With Autism: Diagnosis and Interventions to Meet Their Needs*. NOTES: You may wish to delve deeply into this book, for it contains excellent reference and historical materials, especially on Asperger's autism. I loathed certain parts of the book; it emphasizes too heavily the link between autism and schizophrenia, which is totally inappropriate with regard to Asperger's autism. It downplays Asperger's as a true form of autism, yet claims that "Asperger's Syndrome shares many features with Kanner's autism." This statement is simply not true, and is in fact contradicted later in the book—by the authors themselves. It approaches a point of resentment, the way this book emphasizes the unfounded link between Asperger's autism and psychosis. This from a book written in 1996! My suggestion is to read this book for the resources, and take everything else with a grain of salt—especially all the psychobabble about schizophrenia and psychosis. This book, in fact, is so disturbing in its inaccurate statements that I would even be suspicious of the dates the authors give for events. For example, they give incorrect dates for both Asperger's and Kanner's findings and publications.

Frith, Uta. *Asperger's Syndrome and Autism*. NOTES: A seminal piece and a must-read. Neither here nor in Attwood (below) will you suffer from claims of ridiculous and unfounded links between Asperger's and psychosis or schizophrenia. Neither will you have to endure other idiocies, because Drs. Frith and Attwood are THE modern-day Asperger pioneers.

Attwood, Tony. *Asperger's Syndrome: A Guide*. NOTES: One of the greatest studies of Asperger's autism in children ever to be written. This far exceeds even Dr. Asperger's own observations. All I can say is, order this book while you can still obtain a copy!

Raty, John and Catherine Johnson. *Shadow Syndromes*. NOTES: Resource for learning more about ADHD and all forms of autism. Also, a good book that shows how NOT to approach autism, Tourette Disease, ADHD or OCD. It is full of stupid errors and lousy comparisons. This is the infamous "addiction" book, in which the good doctors claim that all the diseases are really addictions. Beware, too, of the included case studies, for they represent the authors' interpretations of events, and not true medical case study results.

Jacobs, Frank. *The Mad World of William M. Gaines*. NOTES: Hilarious and penetrating look at the founder of "Mad Magazine," and an excellent study of mild Asperger's autism and OCB. In fact this biography far outstrips Ledgin's book in the subject of identifying telltale signs of mild autism.

Vallentin, Antonina. *The Drama of Albert Einstein*. NOTES: Though this excellent 1954 big-hit biography was censured by Einstein himself, who went as far as calling Ms. Vallentin a liar, it is well known that she was indeed a close family friend for decades. Her descriptions of Einstein's autistic behavior, and her unabashed love for him, are what ultimately made her an enemy of the Einstein family. This is a must-read, whether for the autistic information or simply for the pleasure of reading an excellent contempo Einstein biography.

Sayen, Jamie. *Einstein In America*. NOTES: Again, another beautifully written biography that penetrates to the heart of its subject. Though Sayen focuses on Einstein's conscience during the atomic age and his life in America, he, too, describes clearly and concisely the autistic symptoms Einstein suffered. Also, like Vallentin's biography, it contains fantastic, never-before-seen photos.

Clark, Ronald. *The Life and Times of Albert Einstein*. NOTES: No one who studies Einstein seriously can miss having this biography on the bookshelf. This is the original definitive Einstein biography, and offers some of the most detailed descriptions of Einstein's autism. Happily, it has been solidly in print since first publication, and is easily attainable in paperback from at any good bookshop.

Michelmore, Peter. *Albert Einstein*. NOTES: This excellent little book, so rare that it is almost impossible to prove it was even published, can be obtained through rare/used book dealers. It is at once simple, direct and charming—and again, illustrates exquisite examples of Einstein's autistic behavior.

Hoffman, Banesh. *Albert Einstein: Creator and Rebel*. NOTES: Though perhaps not the largest or most impressive Einstein biography, Hoffman, a co-worker of Einstein's, leads us into the world of Einstein's Tourettic behavior as well as the autistic. Hoffman is more interested here in peeling away the layers of Einstein's thought processes—a dream he was ultimately unable to attain.

Paradi , Valerie. *Elijah's Cup: A Family's Journey into the Community and Culture of High-Functioning Autism and Asperger's Syndrome*. NOTES: Though a fascinating story of a mother who claims to suffer from a "shadow" of her son's autism, and her son's struggles to connect with the world, I would not highly recommend this book. It is filled with clumsy and careless factual errors (for example, the author persists in confusing echolalia with palilalia). At times it leans a little too heavily toward the author rather than the subject; still, this book is a deeply personal, almost sensual dive into the world of a lone mother raising a very delicate, wonderful autistic boy. Beware, too, of the almost Munchausen-by-proxy undertones evidenced in the author's prose; she seems more interested in herself and her autobiography than in her son. I'd like to note here that this book reminds me of Lowell Handler's alleged Tourette Syndrome book, Twist and Shout. The book has nothing to do with TS and everything to do with being a Lowell Handler autobiography. What's sad about Handler's book is that it is not even a good autobio. It is so repulsive an attempt at fame-grabbing that I do not have it otherwise listed in this bibliography. (No one should list it in any bibliography.)

Wallace, Amy. *The Prodigy*. NOTES: This is the only (and definitive) biography of child prodigy Bill Sidis. Though Wallace does an exquisite job of illuminating Sidis' later life, and quotes extensively from pertinent and interesting documents, she is rather heavy in some chapters on unnecessary details. Aside from this padding, the book is really one of the best biographies to have around if you are interested in autism and intelligence, or simply fascinated by the links between autism, genius and child prodigies. Wallace does a nice job of slipping in a biographical cameo and several quotes of Norbert Wiener, another great autistic geniurs and Harvard classmate of Sidis'. Wallace reminds us of the "Sidis Fallacy," a psychological term indicating that pressure placed on gifted children will backfire in later life. I.e., Einstein's family raised him contrary to the Sidis Fallacy.

FILMS/PROGRAMS/VIDEOS:

The Mind Traveler with Oliver Sacks: A Rage for Order. Public Broadcasting Station documentary about autism, 1999. NOTES: This penetrating look at autism (and Sacks' thinking processes) is an absolute must-see. In it, he concentrates on Jesse Parks, the famous autistic artist who is also the subject of a book written by her own mother. I do not know if these programs are available on video—Dr. Sacks did two series of them, one for America and an earlier one for Britain. Dr. Sacks' website can always be consulted. Who knows—he may respond to you in person, as he did to me.

Thelonious Monk: Straight, No Chaser. Dir. Charlotte Zwerin. Prod. Clint Eastwood. Documentary, 1988, re-issue 1997. NOTES: An excellent view of Tourette symptoms as well as autism. Excerpts of this film were featured in Polly Draper's "The Tic Code." Most of the footage of Monk, thought for decades to have been destroyed or lost, is excellent and clear—a fascinating look, also, at a period in history and its central figure that changed America forever. No raining-on-your-parade intended, but you will find this marvelous, historic video IMPOSSIBLE to find, unless your rare video dealer or local library happen to own a copy.

I welcome correspondence from anyone interested in Tourette Syndrome, Asperger's Syndrome, autism, Obsessive Compulsive Disease, synesthesia… and bowties!

MOST REVEREND ANTONIO HERNANDEZ
UNIPHYSITE BUDDHIST ORDER
2118 MORTON DRIVE
EAST MOLINE IL 61244
E-mail: suriak@yahoo.com

Printed in the United States
1507400004B/220-222